P9-DUB-305

Evaluation & Management of

Obesity

Evaluation & Management of Obesity

Daniel H. Bessesen, MD
Associate Professor
Division of Endocrinology, Department of Medicine
University of Colorado Health Sciences Center
Chief of Endocrinology
Denver Health Medical Center
Denver, Colorado

Robert Kushner, MD
Professor
Department of Medicine
Northwestern University Medical School
Medical Director, Wellness Institute
Northwestern Memorial Hospital
Chicago, Illinois

From the Centers for Obesity Research and Education

Hanley & Belfus, Inc. / Philadelphia

Publisher: HANLEY & BELFUS. INC.
Medical Publishers
210 South 13th Street
Philadelphia, PA 19107
(215) 546-7293; 800-962-1892
FAX (215) 790-9330
Web site: http://www.hanleyandbelfus.com

Note to the reader: Although the information in this book has been carefully reviewed for correctness of dosage and indications, neither the authors nor the editors nor the publisher can accept any legal responsibility for any errors or omissions that may be made. Neither the publisher nor the editors make any warranty, expressed or implied, with respect to the material contained herein. Before prescribing any drug, the reader must review the manufacturer's current product information (package inserts) for accepted indications, absolute dosage recommendations, and other information pertinent to the safe and effective use of the product described.

Library of Congress Cataloging-in-Publication Data

Evaluation and management of obesity / edited by Daniel Bessesen, Robert F. Kushner.
      p. ; cm.
   Includes bibliographical references.
   ISBN 1-56053-469-9 (alk. paper)
   1. Obesity—Handbooks, manuals, etc. I. Bessesen, Daniel, 1956- II. Kushner,
Robert F., 1953-
   [DNLM: 1. Obesity—prevention & control. 2. Obesity—therapy. WD 210 E917
   2001]
RC628 .E92 2001
616.3'98—dc21

                                                                    2001039936

EVALUATION AND MANAGEMENT OF OBESITY   ISBN -56053-469-9

© 2002 by Hanley & Belfus, Inc. All rights reserved. No part of this book may be reproduced, reused, republished, or transmitted in any form, or stored in a data base or retrieval system, without written permission of the publisher.

Last digit is the print number: 9   8   7   6   5   4   3   2   1

Dedication

We would like to dedicate this book to our wives, Mary and Nancy, and to our children, Max and Anna (DB), and Sarah and Steve (RK). They are the source of the greatest joy in our lives. They have been patient with our late evenings at the computer and our absences from home as we try to teach and learn from other health care providers regarding the treatment of obese people.

Contents

Contributors

Amy C. Baltes, R.D., L.D.
Nutrition and Exercise Specialist, Wellness Institute, Northwestern Memorial Hospital, Chicago, Illinois

Daniel H. Bessesen, M.D.
Associate Professor, Division of Endrocrinology, Department of Medicine, University of Colorado Health Sciences Center; Chief of Endocrinology, Denver Health Medical Center, Denver, Colorado

Susan Bowerman, M.S., R.D.
Assistant Director, UCLA Center for Human Nutrition, UCLA Medical Center, Los Angeles, California

Morgan Downey, J.D.
Executive Director, American Obesity Association, Washington, D.C.

Gary D. Foster, Ph.D.
Associate Professor, Department of Psychiatry, Clinical Director, Weight and Eating Disorders Program, University of Pennsylvania School of Medicine, Philadelphia, Pennsylvania

Kara Gallagher, Ph.D.
Research Associate, Weight Control and Diabetes Research Center, The Miriam Hospital, Providence, Rhode Island

David Heber, M.D., Ph.D.
Professor of Medicine and Public Health, UCLA Center for Human Nutrition, UCLA Medical Center, Los Angeles, California

James O. Hill, Ph.D.
Professor, Department of Pediatrics, Director, Center for Human Nutrition, University of Colorado Health Sciences Center, Denver, Colorado

Dawn Jackson, R.D., L.D.
Nutrition and Exercise Specialist, Wellness Institute, Northwestern Memorial Hospital, Chicago, Illinois

John Jackicic, Ph.D.
Associate Professor, Weight Control and Diabetes Research Center, Brown Medical School, The Miriam Hospital, Providence, Rhode Island

Robert Kushner, M.D.
Professor, Department of Medicine, Northwestern University Medical School,
Medical Director, Wellness Institute, Northwestern Memorial Hospital,
Chicago, Illinois

John C. Peters, Ph.D.
Associate Director, Food and Beverage Technology, Procter and Gamble,
Cincinnati, Ohio

Laura Primak, R.D., C.S.P., C.N.S.D.
Nutritionist, Nutrition Academic Award Program, Department of Pediatrics,
University of Colorado Health Sciences Center, Denver, Colorado

Thomas Robinson, M.D., M.P.H.
Assistant Professor, Department of Pediatrics, Center for Research in Disease
Prevention, Department of Medicine, Stanford University School of Medicine,
Stanford, California; Division of General Pediatrics, Lucile Packard Children's
Hospital at Stanford, and Stanford Univeristy Hospital, Palo Alto, California

Rena R. Wing, Ph.D.
Professor of Psychiatry and Human Behavior, Brown University School of
Medicine, The Miriam Hospital, Providence, Rhode Island

Holly R. Wyatt, M.D.
Assistant Professor, Division of Endocrinology, Metabolism, and Diabetes,
Department of Medicine, University of Colorado Health Sciences Center,
Denver, Colorado

Preface

Obesity is a frustrating problem to have (for the patient) and to treat (by the physician). It appears to be a root cause of many of the most common health problems in the United States, and it is increasing in prevalence and incidence around the world. In this book, we have asked a number of the most experienced clinician/investigators in the country to provide the insights that they have gained from years of treating overweight and obese patients. The result is not so much a "consensus guide" to treatment, but rather a look at the clinical framework that guides the practice of experienced clinicians in the treatment of the obese patient. We hope that this guide will provide practical, immediately useful strategies and tools to primary care physicians, subspecialty fellows, house officers, medical students and all health professionals who feel inadequately prepared to care for obese patients. We also hope that it will provide some new information to experienced clinicians who wish to broaden their repertoire of strategies.

Our goal from the outset was to provide a balanced view of controversies in specific treatment approaches in the management of obesity, attempting to neither overstate nor understate the potential benefits and risks.

We are deeply indebted to the tremendous group of contributing authors who took time from their busy schedules to share their thoughts and experience with all of us. Many of the contributing authors come from the Centers for Obesity Research and Education, or C.O.R.E. C.O.R.E. consists of 8 nationally recognized centers involved with the medical management of overweight and obese persons in the United States. It is organized around a unified goal to disseminate knowledge about obesity management to the medical community. The list of sites, their directors, coordinators, and contact information is listed below. C.O.R.E. sponsors educational programs on obesity treatment throughout the year. Information on educational programs in your area can be found on the C.O.R.E. website at www.uchsc.edu/core/. C.O.R.E. receives financial support from a number of companies interested in obesity treatment, but these sponsors have had no input into the content of this book.

Perhaps most importantly, we acknowledge our debt to the many overweight and obese patients who have shared with us the wealth of their individual lives, the burden of their illness, and their own experiences of treatment. These people have been our best teachers.

Daniel H. Bessesen, MD
Robert Kushner, MD

C.O.R.E. Contact List

Northwestern Memorial Wellness Institute
Principal: Robert Kushner, MD
Coordinator: Leigh Ginther
240 E. Ontario, Ste. 400, Chicago, IL 60611. Phone: (312) 926-8895,
Fax: (312) 503-2123; E-mail: lginther@nmh.org

Pennington Biomedical Research Center
Principals: George Bray, MD, Donna Ryan, MD
Coordinator: Eleanor Meador, RN
Louisiana State University, Pennington Biomedical Research Center, 6400
Perkins Road, Baton Rouge, LA 70808-4124
Phone: (225) 763-2529, Fax: (225) 763-2525,
E-mail: meadoreh@mhs.pbrc.edu

St. Luke's–Roosevelt Hospital Center
Principals: Xavier Pi-Sunyer, MD, Cathy Nonas, MS, RD, CDE
Coordinator: Betty Kovacs, MS, RD
St. Luke's–Roosevelt Hospital Center, VanItallie Center, 425 West 59th St.,
#9D, New York, NY 10019
Phone: (212) 523-8440, Fax: (212) 523-8103; E-mail: BLK916@aol.com,
Pager: (917) 960-5064

UCLA
Principal: Dave Heber, MD, PhD
Coordinator: Susan Bowerman, MS, RD
UCLA Center for Human Nutrition, Warren Hall, Rm. 12-217, 900 Veterans
Avenue, Los Angeles, CA 90095-1742
Phone: (310) 206-1987, Fax: (310) 206-5264, E-mail:
sbowerman@mednet.ucla.edu

University of Colorado Health Sciences Center—Coordinating Center
Program Director: Holly Wyatt, MD
Principals: James O. Hill, PhD, Dan Bessesen, MD
Coordinator: Bonnie Jortberg, MS, RD, CDE
University of Colorado Health Sciences Center, 4200 E. 9th Ave., Campus Box
C-225, Denver, CO 80262
Phone: (303) 315-0123, Fax: (303) 315-3273, E-mail:
bonnie.jortberg@uchsc.edu

Beth Israel Deaconess Medical Center
Principals: George Blackburn, MD, PhD, Carolina Apovian, MD, FACN
Coordinator: Susan Morreale, CHES

332 Washington Street, Suite 360, Wellesley Hills, MA 02481
Phone: (781) 431-2627, Fax: (781) 431-2647, E-mail:
neche2@mindspring.com

Mayo Clinic
Principal: Michael Jensen, MD
Coordinator: Ms. Kelly Dunagan
Mayo Clinic, Dept. of Endocrinology, Metabolism and Nutrition, 2000 1st
Street, SW, West 18, Rochester, MN 55905
Phone: (507) 538-1565, Fax: (507) 284-5745, E-mail:
dunagan.kelly@mayo.edu

Minnesota Obesity Center
Principal: Charles Billington, MD
Coordinator: Heidi Hoover, MS, RD
VA Medical Center, Nutrition Section, 1 Veterans Drive, Mail Code 120,
Minneapolis, MN 55417
Phone: (612) 725-2004, Fax: (612) 727-5997, E-mail:
hoover.heidi@med.va.gov

Chapter 1

Robert Kushner, MD

Defining the Scope of the Problem of Obesity

If you are like other physicians, you are seeing more obese patients in your practice than ever before. The reason is that, for the first time in history, a majority of American adults are overweight. According to the 1999 statistics from the Centers for Disease Control and Prevention (CDC), 61% of U.S. adults are now considered overweight. More than a third of adults, 35%, are slightly or moderately overweight (defined as a body mass index [BMI] 25 to 29.9), and more than a quarter of Americans, 26%, are considered obese (BMI 30.0 or higher). For comparison, only 43% of the population was overweight between 1960-62. The statistics are even more disturbing for minority women, where the age-specific prevalence of each level of overweight and obesity is higher for non-Hispanic black women (66.5%) and for Mexican-American women (67.6%) than for white women (45.5%), according to the 1988-94 survey. For children aged 6 to 17 years, the prevalence of overweight has risen from about 4% in 1963 to over 10% by 1994. We also know that the prevalence of overweight and obesity tends to rise with advancing age until ages 50 to 60 years old. This modern-day public health epidemic represents one of the most important contributors to increased morbidity, mortality, and healthcare expenditures in America.

And we are not alone. The prevalence of overweight is also rising to epidemic proportions in other "westernized" and less developed countries around the world. In Russia, the figure is 54%; in the United Kingdom 51%; and in Germany 50%. Fifteen percent of China's adult population is now considered overweight. According to the Report of a World Health Organization (WHO) Consultation on Obesity, "overweight and obesity are now so common that they are replacing the more traditional public health concerns such as undernutrition and infectious diseases as some of the most significant contributors to ill health."

You can think of overweight as an unintended consequence of modern society. Its etiology is multifactorial, presumably brought about by an interaction between predisposing genetic and metabolic factors and a rapidly changing environment. Interactive influences include social, behavioral, physiological, and metabolic factors. By simple definition, obesity is a disease of energy imbalance, where "energy in" exceeds "energy out." The societal pressures that expose individuals to high-calorie, high-fat convenience foods along with technical advances that promote sedentary behavior have led to involuntary obesity. These social and environmental causes of an energy imbalance are considered the major underlying factors for the markedly increased prevalence of obesity over the past several decades. The WHO recently concluded that the fundamental causes of the obesity epidemic worldwide are a fall in spontaneous and work-related physical activity and over-consumption of high-fat, energy-dense diets. These two principal factors tend to overwhelm an individual's normal physiologic adjustments in food intake and metabolism in order to maintain normal energy balance. Attention to these remedial environmental factors forms the cornerstone of obesity treatment.

Insights into the genetic and metabolic control systems that govern regulation of body weight have exploded over the past 7 years. The landmark discovery of the ob gene and its protein product, leptin (from the Greek work *leptos*, meaning "thin"), in 1994 opened the way for further understanding of how mammals sense the amount of adipose tissue stored in the body and compensate for energy imbalance. It appears that multiple feedback loops exist between the central and autonomic nervous systems, the endocrine glands, and adipose tissue that operate to adjust hunger, satiety, and energy expenditure (see chapter 21). Although the precise mechanisms are uncertain, it is thought that about 25 to 40% of individual differences in body weight depend on genetic factors. Further elucidation of the intricacies of the metabolic regulatory system should pave the way for discovery of new pharmacologic treatment approaches. In summary, both environment and genetics play a role in whether an individual will be overweight and in the potential severity of the weight gain.

The greatest concern of the obesity epidemic is the effect on patients' health. Obesity, along with diet and physical inactivity, is responsible for approximately 300,000 preventable deaths per year. Only cigarette smoking ranks higher as a public health concern. Obesity is linked to the most prevalent and costly medical problems seen in our country, including type 2 diabetes, hypertension, coronary artery disease, and some forms of cancer. Table 1 estimates the proportion of disease prevalence attributable to obesity. Although these figures are difficult to calculate and subject to variation, it is

TABLE 1. Proportion of Disease Prevalence Attributable to Obesity

Type 2 diabetes	57%
Hypertension	17%
Coronary heart disease	17%
Gallbladder disease	30%
Osteoarthritis	14%
Breast cancer	11%
Uterine cancer	11%
Colon cancer	11%

estimated that 57% of type 2 diabetes is directly attributable to underlying obesity, as is 17% of hypertension and coronary artery disease; 11% of breast, uterine and colon cancer; 14% of osteoarthritis; and 30% of gallbladder disease. In other words, if obesity could be controlled, the prevalence of these (and other) diseases would be expected to fall by the respective percentages. In total, obesity affects at least nine organ systems. Table 2 lists the symptoms and diseases that are directly or indirectly related to obesity. Although individuals will vary, the number and severity of organ specific co-morbidities usually rises with increasing levels of obesity.

TABLE 2. Disorders and Symptoms Related to Obesity

• **Cardiovascular**	• **Respiratory**
Hypertension	Dyspnea and Fatigue
Congestive Heart Failure	Obstructive Sleep Apnea
Cor Pulmonale	Hypoventilation Syndrome
Varicose Veins	Pickwickian Syndrome
Pulmonary Embolism	• **Endocrine**
Coronary Artery Disease	Insulin resistance (Syndrome X)
• **Neurologic**	Type 2 diabetes
Stroke	Dyslipidemia
Idiopathic intracranial hypertension	Polycystic ovarian syndrome (PCOS)/
Meralgia paresthetica	hyperandrogenism (F)
• **Musculoskeletal**	Amenorrhea/infertility
Immobility	• **Gastrointestinal**
Degenerative arthritis	Gastroesophageal reflux disease (GERD)
Low back pain	Hepatic steatosis
• **Integument**	Non-alcoholic steatohepatitis (NASH)
Venous stasis of legs	Cholelithiasis
Cellulitis	Hernias
Diminished hygiene	Colon cancer
Intertrigo, carbuncles	• **Genitourinary**
• **Psychological**	Urinary stress incontinence
Depression/low self-esteem	Hypogonadism (M)
BED	Breast and uterine cancer

Obesity is a chronic, life-long disease that warrants action. The disease is spreading across the globe with America as the epicenter. It is likely that today's overweight children will be tomorrow's obese adults. This is a cycle that will continue unless we employ broad-based public health initiatives and target high-risk individuals for weight management. We hope that this book provides you with some useful tools in your work with overweight and obese patients.

References

1. World Health Organization: Preventing and Managing the Global Epidemic of Obesity. Report of the WHO Consultation on Obesity. WHO, 1997.

2. Flegal KM, Carroll MD, Kuczmarski RJ, Johnson CL: Overweight and obesity in the United States: prevalence and trends, 1960-1994. Int J Obesity 1998;22:39-47.
3. Mokdad AH, Bowman BA, Ford ES, Vinicor F, Marks JS, Koplan JP: The continuing epidemics of obesity and diabetes in the United States. JAMA 2001;286: 1195-1200.
4. Must A, Spadano J, Coakley E, Field A, Colditz G, Dietz W: The disease burden associated with overweight and obesity. JAMA 1999;282:1523-1529.
5. National Task Force on the Prevention and Treatment of Obesity: Overweight, obesity, and health risk. Arch Intern Med 2000;160:898-904.

Chapter 2

Robert Kushner, MD

Office-based Obesity Care: Setting Up the Office Environment

One of the most significant obstacles to obesity care during a routine office visit is availability of time. Recent surveys show that the average length of an office visit is less than 20 minutes. Within these confines, the physician typically elicits a brief history, performs a limited physical examination, reviews and interprets pertinent laboratory and diagnostic tests, and provides recommendations that may include ordering further tests, writing prescriptions, and conducting counseling. Accordingly, care of the obese patient (and all patients) would be greatly facilitated by incorporating efficient and effective office-based systems. Table 1 lists the office-based systems that are uniquely geared to the care of the obese patient. Collectively, they address a need for heightened sensitivity and thoroughness throughout all office systems.

■ The Physical Environment

Accessibility to the office is critical for the obese patient. Facility limitations include difficult access from the parking lot or stairs, narrow doors and hallways, and cramped restrooms. One of the first concerns obese patients have upon entering the waiting room is where they can safely sit. Office chairs with standard width and side arm rests will not comfortably accommodate moderately to severely obese patients. Ideal chairs have no arms, so that patients do not have to squeeze themselves into predefined "normal" dimensions.

■ Equipment

Accurate measurement of height and weight is paramount to treating patients with obesity. All too often, the physician's office has a scale that does not measure above 350 pounds, or the foot platform is too narrow to securely balance the overweight individual. Although a wall-mounted sliding statiometer is the most accurate instrument, a sturdy height meter attached to the scale will suffice. The weight scale should preferably have a wide base with a nearby handle bar for support if necessary. Depending on the patient population, it is reasonable to select a scale that measures in excess of 350 pounds. To protect privacy, the scale should be located in a private area of the office.

TABLE 1. Office-based Obesity Care

The Physical Environment
    Accessibility and comfort: Stairs, doorways, hallways, restrooms, waiting-room chairs and space, reading materials, and other educational materials

Equipment
    Large adult and thigh blood pressure cuffs, large gowns, step stools, adequate weight and height scales, and tape measure

Materials
    Educational and behavior-promoting handouts on diet, exercise, medications, surgery, BMI, and obesity-associated diseases

Tools
    Previsit questionnaires, BMI stamps, food and activity diaries, and pedometers

Protocols
    Patient care treatment protocols for return visit schedule, medications, and referrals to dietitians and psychologists

Staffing
    Team approach to include office nurse, physician assistant, nurse practitioner, and health advocate

Examination rooms should have large gowns available as well as a step stool to mount the examination tables. Each room should be equipped with large adult and thigh blood pressure cuffs. A cuff bladder that is too small will overestimate the pressure and lead to a false diagnosis of hypertension. To avoid errors, the bladder width should be 40 to 50% of upper-arm circumference. Therefore, a large adult cuff (15 cm wide) should be chosen for patients with mild to moderate obesity while a thigh cuff (18 cm wide) should be used for patients whose arm circumferences are greater than 16 inches. A cloth or metal tape should be available for measurement of waist circumference as per the NHLBI Practical Guide for obesity classification.

■ Using an Integrated Team Approach

How practices operate on a day-to-day basis is extremely important for effective obesity care. Several key office-based strategies have been shown to improve practice performance in relation to goals for primary care. Two of the most successful features are use of a multidisciplinary or interdisciplinary team and incorporation of protocols and procedures. Because of limited time, physicians are generally unable to provide all of the care necessary for treatment. Moreover, other personnel are often better qualified to deliver dietary, physical activity, and behavioral counseling. Accordingly, there is an opportunity for other office staff to play a greater role in the care of obese patients. A sense of "groupness," defined as the degree to which the group practice identifies itself and functions as a team, will enhance the quality and efficiency of care.

The optimal team composition and management structure will vary between practices. As an example, receptionists can provide information about the program, including general philosophy, staffing, fee schedules, and other written materials; registered nurses can obtain vital measurements, including height and weight (for body mass index) and waist circumference, and instruct on and review food and activity journals and other educational materials; and physician assistants can monitor the progress of treatment and assume many of the other responsibilities of care. Regardless of how the work load is delegated, the physician should be perceived as the team leader and source of common philosophy of care.

■ Protocols and Procedures

The time spent in the evaluation and treatment of the obese patient can be enhanced by use of protocols and procedures. A self-administered medical history questionnaire can be either mailed to the patient prior to the initial visit or completed in the waiting room. In addition to standard questions, sections of the form should inquire about past obesity treatment programs, a body weight history, current diet and physical activity levels, social support, and goals and expectations. The review-of-systems section can include medical prompts that are more commonly seen among the obese, such as snoring, morning headaches and daytime sleepiness (for obstructive sleep apnea), urinary incontinence, intertrigo, and sexual dysfunction, among others.

Identifying the body mass index (BMI) as a fifth vital sign may also increase physician awareness and prompt counseling. Use of prompts, alerts, or other reminders have been shown to significantly increase physician performance of other health maintenance activities. Once the patient is identified as overweight or obese, printed food and activity diaries and patient information sheets on a variety of topics such as the food-guide pyramid, deciphering food labels, healthy snacking, dietary fiber, aerobic exercise and resistance training, and dealing with stress can be used to support behavior change and facilitate patient education. Ready-to-copy materials can be obtained from a variety of sources for free or a minimal fee. Finally, protocols and procedures for various treatment pathways can be established for obtaining periodic laboratory monitoring and referral to allied health professionals, such as registered dietitians, exercise specialists, and clinical psychologists.

Attention to the office environment and staff is an important feature of successful obesity care. Take time to review your practice and use Table 1 as a check list to survey office-based systems.

References

1. Mechanic D, McAlpine DD, Rosenthal M: Are patients' office visits with physicians getting shorter? N Engl J Med 2001;344:198-204.
2. Stange KC, Zyzanski SJ, Jaen CR, et al: Illuminating the 'black box'. A description of 4454 patient visits to 138 family physicians. J Fam Prac 1998;46: 377-389.

3. 10 Steps: Implementation Guide. Put Prevention into Practice. Adapted from The Clinicians' Handbook of Preventive Services, 2nd Edition, Publication No. 98-0025, 1998. Agency for Healthcare Research and Quality, Rockville, MD. http://www.ahrq.gov/ppip/impsteps.htm

4. Yano EM, Fink A, Hirsch SH, Robbins AS, Rubenstein LV: Helping practices reach primary care goals. Lessons from the literature. Arch Intern Med 1995; 155:1146-1156.

5. Kushner R, Pendarvis L: An integrated approach to obesity care. Nutr Clin Care 1999;2:285-291.

6. Frank A: A multidisciplinary approach to obesity management: The physician's role and team care alternatives. J Am Diet Assoc 1998;98(Suppl 2):S44-S48.

7. Crabtree BF, Miller WL, Aita VA, Flocke SA, Stange KC: Primary care practice organization and preventive services delivery: A qualitative analysis. J Fam Pract 1998;46:404-409.

8. Scholle SH, Agatisa PK, Krohn MA, Johnson J, McLaughlin MK: Locating a health advocate in a private obstetrics/gynecology office increases patient's receipt of preventive recommendations. J Women's Health & Gender-Based Medicine 2000;9:161-165.

9. Balas EA, Weingarten S, Garb CT, Blumenthal D, Boren SA, Brown GD: Improving preventive care by prompting physicians. Arch Intern Med 2000; 160:301-308.

10. Kreuter MW, Chheda SG, Bull FC: How does physician advice influence patient behavior? Evidence for a priming effect. Arch Fam Med 2000;9:426-433.

11. Swinburn BA, Walter LG, Arroll B, Tilyard MW, Russell DG: The green prescription study: A randomized controlled trial of written advice provided by general practitioners. Am J Public Health 1998;88:288-291.

12. Albright CL, Cohen S, Gibbons L, Miller S, Marcus B, Sallis J, et al: Incorporating physical activity advice into primary care. Physician-delivered advice within the activity counseling trial. Am J Prev Med 2000;18:225-234.

Chapter 3

Daniel H. Bessesen, MD

Medical Evaluation of the Overweight or Obese Patient

■ Measuring the Degree of Obesity

Once the decision is made to evaluate and treat obese patients as a routine part of office care, it may be useful to optimize systems in the office to make this process easier. Observe what happens in the waiting room and at the front desk to see how the office staff can help with these patients (see chapter 2). In addition to having an office that is "friendly" to obese patients, the check-in procedures should include measures that will help assess the degree of obesity present in these patients. Although there are a variety of methods available for determining body fat content (see chapter 4), in general clinical practice the two most useful methods are calculating the body mass index (BMI) and measuring the waist circumference. BMI is calculated as the weight in kilograms divided by the height in meters squared. The easiest way to determine the BMI of an individual patient is to use a table which converts height in inches and weight in pounds into a value for BMI (Table 1). The BMI allows classification of patients as to degree of obesity (Table 2). The more severe the obesity, the more aggressive evaluation and treatment should be. Consider having a BMI poster near the scales used to weigh patients, and having the office staff educate patients about the meaning of the BMI.

The body mass index has some limitations. In younger individuals who are muscular or older individuals with edema, the BMI may overestimate fat mass. In those who have lost lean body mass, especially elderly individuals, the BMI may underestimate body fat. There are ways to overcome this problem. Considering that BMI attempts to assess the health risks associated with body weight, recent evidence suggests that the single best predictor of adverse health effects from excess body fat is visceral adiposity (i.e., the adipose tissue contained within the abdominal cavity). One way to estimate visceral adiposity is the waist circumference. The method used to measure waist circumference is depicted in Figure 1. Place the tape measure either between the iliac crest and the lower rib cage or at the level of the iliac crest, parallel to the floor, and measure the circumference at the end of a relaxed exhalation. A high-risk waist circumference in men is greater then 40 inches (>102 cm), or greater than 35 inches (>85 cm) in women. Measuring the waist circumference is most useful in those individuals with a body mass

TABLE 1. Body Mass Index Table

BMI Height (inches)	19	20	21	22	23	24	25	26	27	28	29	30	31	32	33	34	35
								Body Weight (pounds)									
58	91	96	100	105	110	115	119	124	129	134	138	143	148	153	158	162	167
59	94	99	104	109	114	119	124	128	133	138	143	148	153	158	163	168	173
60	97	102	107	112	118	123	128	133	138	143	148	153	158	163	168	174	179
61	100	106	111	116	122	127	132	137	143	148	153	158	164	169	174	180	185
62	104	109	115	120	126	131	136	142	147	153	158	164	169	175	180	186	191
63	107	113	118	124	130	135	141	146	152	158	163	169	175	180	186	191	197
64	110	116	122	128	134	140	145	151	157	163	169	174	180	186	192	197	204
65	114	120	126	132	138	144	150	156	162	168	174	180	186	192	198	204	210
66	118	124	130	136	142	148	155	161	167	173	179	186	192	198	204	210	216
67	121	127	134	140	146	153	159	166	172	178	185	191	198	204	211	217	223
68	125	131	138	144	151	158	164	171	177	184	190	197	203	210	216	223	230
69	128	135	142	149	155	162	169	176	182	189	196	203	209	216	223	230	236
70	132	139	146	153	160	167	174	181	188	195	202	209	216	222	229	236	243
71	136	143	150	157	165	172	179	186	193	200	208	215	222	229	236	243	250
72	140	147	154	162	169	177	184	191	199	206	213	221	228	235	242	250	258
73	144	151	159	166	174	182	189	197	204	212	219	227	235	242	250	257	265
74	148	155	163	171	179	186	194	202	210	218	225	233	241	249	256	264	272
75	152	160	168	176	184	192	200	208	216	224	232	240	248	256	264	272	279
76	156	164	172	180	189	197	205	213	221	230	238	246	254	263	271	279	287

BMI	36	37	38	39	40	41	42	43	44	45	46	47	48	49	50	51	52	53	54
Height (inches)									Body Weight (pounds)										
58	172	177	181	186	191	196	201	205	210	215	220	224	229	234	239	244	248	253	258
59	178	183	188	193	198	203	208	212	217	222	227	232	237	242	247	252	257	262	267
60	184	189	194	199	204	209	215	220	225	230	235	240	245	250	255	261	266	271	276
61	190	195	201	206	211	217	222	227	232	238	243	248	254	259	264	269	275	280	285
62	196	202	207	213	218	224	229	235	240	246	251	256	262	267	273	278	284	289	295
63	203	208	214	220	225	231	237	242	248	254	259	265	270	278	282	287	293	299	304
64	209	215	221	227	232	238	244	250	256	262	267	273	279	285	291	296	302	308	314
65	216	222	228	234	240	246	252	258	264	270	276	282	288	294	300	306	312	318	324
66	223	229	235	241	247	253	260	266	272	278	284	291	297	303	309	315	322	328	334
67	230	236	242	249	255	261	268	274	280	287	293	299	306	312	319	325	331	338	344
68	236	243	249	256	262	269	276	282	289	295	302	308	315	322	328	335	341	348	354
69	243	250	257	263	270	277	284	291	297	304	311	318	324	331	338	345	351	358	365
70	250	257	264	271	278	285	292	299	306	313	320	327	334	341	348	355	362	369	376
71	257	265	272	279	286	293	301	308	315	322	329	338	343	351	358	365	372	379	386
72	265	272	279	287	294	302	309	316	324	331	338	346	353	361	368	375	383	390	397
73	272	280	288	295	302	310	318	325	333	340	348	355	363	371	378	386	393	401	408
74	280	287	295	303	311	319	326	334	342	350	358	365	373	381	389	396	404	412	420
75	287	295	303	311	319	327	335	343	351	359	367	375	383	391	399	407	415	423	431
76	295	304	312	320	328	336	344	353	361	369	377	385	394	402	410	418	426	435	443

TABLE 2. Classification of Overweight and Obesity by BMI, Waist Circumference, and Associated Disease Risk*

	BMI (kg/m2)	Obesity Class	Disease Risk* (Relative to Normal Weight and Waist Circumference) Men ≤40 in (≤ 102 cm) Women ≤ 35 in (≤ 88 cm)	Men > 40 in (> 102 cm) Women > 35 in (≥ 88 cm)
Underweight	< 18.5		—	—
Normal†	18.5–24.9		—	—
Overweight	25.0–29.9		Increased	High
Obesity	30.0–34.9	I	High	Very High
	35.0–39.9	II	Very High	Very High
Extreme Obesity	≥ 40	III	Extremely High	Extremely High

*Disease risk for type 2 dibetes, hypertension, and CVD.

†Increased waist circumference can also be a marker for increased risk even in persons of normal weight.

Adapted from "Preventing and Managing the Global Epidemic of Obesity. Report of the World Health Organization Consultation of Obesity." WHO, Geneva, June 1997.

index between 25 and 35. For example, if a 27-year-old man presents with a measured BMI of 28 (overweight) and a lot of muscle mass is observed, then a waist circumference less than 40 inches is reassuring that his slightly increased BMI is not predictive of adverse health affects. Conversely, if a woman presents with a BMI of 29 (overweight) and a waist circumference of 39 inches, treatment is indicated for the risk associated with a BMI in the obese range.

■ Assessing Risk: Beyond BMI and Waist Circumference

The aggressiveness of encouragement offered to an individual patient to manage his or her weight depends on the degree of risk for adverse health consequences. BMI and waist circumference aid in risk stratifying your patients; however, a number of other factors will improve this risk assessment. If an individual already has adverse health problems related to weight, the obesity should be treated more aggressively. If the patient is currently healthy but has a positive family history for adverse health problems including diabetes, coronary artery disease, and hypertension, that patient is at a higher risk for future health problems and deserves more attention. Age also plays a role. As the patient's age increases so does the risk for adverse health consequences. A healthy 25-year-old person with a BMI of 30 is less likely to experience adverse health consequences in the next 5 years as compared to a 40 year-old. This is not to say it is unimportant to prevent complications of

FIGURE 1.

Waist Circumference Measurement

To measure waist circumference, locate the upper hip bone and the top of the right iliac crest. Place a measuring tape in a horizontal plane around the abdomen at the level of the iliac crest. Before reading the tape measure, ensure that the tape is snug, but does not compress the skin, and is parallel to the floor. The measurement is made at the end of a normal expiration.

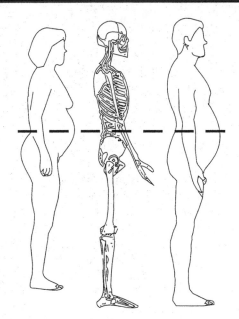

Measuring-Tape Position for Waist (Abdominal) Circumference in Adults

obesity in younger individuals, only that their health risks are somewhat lower. Physical inactivity also increases the risk for adverse health consequences. Overweight individuals in excellent physical condition may actually have a lower absolute risk of health problems than a relatively lean individual who is extremely sedentary (see chapter 12). Part of a health assessment involves asking questions that offer an idea of the patient's usual pattern of physical activity. Finally, consider screening patients for conditions that are associated with or might have contributed to the development of obesity.

■ Screening for Other Diseases

The person who already has adverse health consequences from obesity deserves more aggressive treatment. A number of screening tests should be used to identify diseases that may have developed slowly without patient awareness. In addition, some believe that their weight problem is the result of a hormone imbalance or metabolic disturbance, yet careful medical evaluation of these patients rarely turns up easily reversible causes of their weight problem. It is important to discuss the biologic nature of weight regulation (see Chapter 21) and point out that conditions such as hypothyroidism or Cushing's syndrome rarely cause the type of obesity seen in the general primary care practice. Although both diseases should at least be considered, the history, physical, and laboratory evaluation should focus on identifying complications of obesity. The common complications of obesity include diabetes, hyperlipidemia, obstructive sleep apnea, and hypertension.

Diabetes

Diabetes is present in 5–9% of all adults in this country. The risk of diabetes increases as age and BMI increase (Figure 2). It is more common in ethnic minorities including Native Americans, Africa Americans, and Hispanics. There are three options for screening the obese or overweight patient for diabetes. One approach would be to check a random glucose while they are in the office. A second approach would be to check a glycosylated hemoglobin level. A third approach would be to check a fasting blood glucose level. While a random glucose greater then 200 mg/dl in a symptomatic individual makes the diagnosis of diabetes, it is not clear what level of glucose obtained at a random time effectively rules out diabetes. A blood sugar of 140 to 200 mg/dl is not normal, but neither is diagnostic for diabetes or rules it out. If a random glucose is used as the office screening test, a result between 140 and 200 mg/dl will require further more definitive testing. A glycosylated hemoglobin is an attractive test because it can be drawn without fasting, and gives information about the average glucose level over the last three months. However, there are problems with how the test is done. The same sample of blood sent to five different clinical laboratories will have glycosylated hemoglobin values that vary by as much as 1 to 2 percentage points, because currently, there is no standard method for performing this assay. As a result, the Amer-

FIGURE 2.

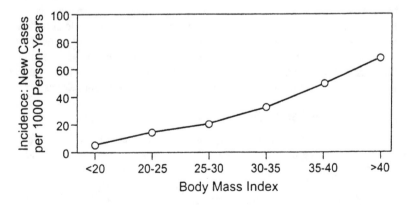

Body mass index and the risk of diabetes. (From Knowler WC, et al: Am J Epidemiol 113:144–156, 1981, with permission.)

ican Diabetes Association does not encourage primary care providers to use this test to diagnose diabetes. However, controversy exists because of the ease and logic of using this test to diagnose diabetes. There are diabetes specialists who think it is an appropriate diagnostic test despite the problems with standardization. If this test is chosen as the standard diagnostic test, the cut-off for diagnosing diabetes should be 1 percentage point above the upper limits of normal for the available assay. The most widely accepted screening and diagnostic test is the fasting plasma glucose. A fasting glucose greater than 126 mg/dl on two occasions in the absence of medical illness establishes a diagnosis of diabetes. Because this test has a high degree of reliability and accuracy, and because it has been extensively studied, this is the preferred method for screening and diagnosis. Fasting plasma glucose levels between 110 and 126 mg/dl are not normal but are not diagnostic of diabetes, and this result would categorize a patient as having impaired glucose tolerance or glucose intolerance. Individuals with this degree of hyperglycemia have an increase risk for coronary artery disease and stroke but are not at risk for microvascular disease.

If an overweight or obese individual is screened and found to have type-2 diabetes, the preferred treatment would probably be metformin as long as the creatinine level is less than 1.3 mg/dl. This medication improves glucose levels without increasing insulin levels. In addition, many patients will not gain or lose weight on this agent. Many practitioners wonder whether it is appropriate to treat individuals with insulin resistance (but not frank diabetes) with metformin or other insulin-sensitizing drugs such as the thiazolidinediones. These ideas are being tested in a number of clinical trials; however, at this point it is probably not indicated. While metformin can cause weight loss and improve glucose tolerance, it is not a very potent weight loss medication. To use a medication to treat weight as well as glucose intolerance, consider a medication that is FDA approved for weight loss (see Chapter 14).

Hypertension

The prevalence of high blood pressure rises as BMI increases (Figure 3), and age advances. Like diabetes, hypertension is more common in African American and Hispanic patients. Overweight and obese individuals should be screened for hypertension like all other adults. It is important that the blood pressure cuff be the appropriate size when taking a measurement in overweight or obese patients. The goals for treatment and medications are no different for an overweight or obese individual than for hypertensive patients of normal weight. However, the presence of hypertension adds another indication for this individual to consider losing weight.

Hyperlipidemia

The presence of obesity is an independent risk factor for coronary artery disease (Figure 4). Adults who are obese should be screened with a fasting lipid panel including measures of total cholesterol, HDL cholesterol, triglyc-

16   Chapter 3

FIGURE 3.

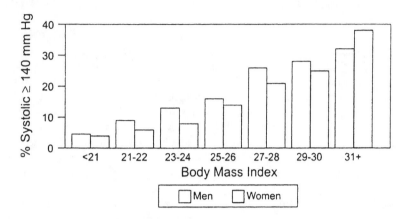

Body mass index and the risk of hypertension. (Canadian Guidelines for Healthy Weights. Cat. no. H39-134 1989E; 1988:69.)

eride, and a calculated value for LDL cholesterol. Treatment of hyperlipidemia should be guided by the recently published National Cholesterol Education Program guidelines (NCEP).[2] Table 3 outlines the major risk factors that the NCEP panel identified as risk factors that modify LDL goals. Table 4 identifies the LDL cholesterol goals for the three categories of risk. Figure 4 from the NCEP guidelines demonstrates the steps to undertake in helping patients modify their lifestyles. Table 5 highlights the medications that are useful in treating hyperlipidemia.

While a patient may present with concerns about their weight, this is an excellent opportunity to consider treatment options with the potential to reduce risk for coronary artery disease. A large number of prospective ran-

**TABLE 3. Major Risk Factors (Exclusive of LDL Cholesterol)
That Modify LDL Goals***

- Cigarette smoking
- Hypertension (blood pressure ≥ 140/90 mm Hg or on antihypertensive medication)
- Low HDL cholesterol (< 40 mg/dL)†
- Family history of premature CHD (CHD in male first-degree relative < 55 years; CHD in female first-degree relative < 65 years)
- Age (men ≥ 45 years; women ≥ 55 years)

*Diabetes is regarded as a coronary heart disease (CHD) risk equivalent. LDL indicates low-density lipoprotein; HDL, high-density lipoprotein.

†HDL cholesterol ≤ 60 mg/dL counts as a "negative" risk factor; its presence removes 1 risk factor from the total count.

TABLE 4. LDL Cholesterol Goals and Cut-off Points for Therapeutic Lifestyle Changes (TLC) and Drug Therapy in Different Risk Categories*

Risk Category	LDL Goal (mg/dL)	LDL Level at Which to Initiate Therapeutic Lifestyle Changes (mg/dL)	LDL Level at Which to Consider Drug Therapy (mg/dL)
CHD or CHD risk equivalents (10-year risk > 20%)	< 100	≥ 100	≥ 130 (100–129: drug optional)†
2+ Risk factors (10-year risk ≥ 20%)	< 130	≥ 130	10-year risk 10%–20%: ≥ 130 10-year risk < 10%: ≥ 160
0–1 Risk factor‡	< 160	≥ 160	≥ 190 (160–189: LDL-lowering drug optional)

*LDL indicates low-density lipoprotein; CHD, coronary heart disease.

†Some authorities recommend use of LDL-lowering drugs in this category if an LDL cholesterol level of <100 mg/dL cannot be achieved by therapeutic lifestyle changes. Others prefer use of drugs that primarily modify triglycerides and HDL, e.g., nicotinic acid or fibrate. Clinical judgment also may call for deferring drug therapy in this subcategory.

‡Almost all people with 0–1 risk factor have a 10-year risk < 10%; thus, 10-year risk assessment in people with 0–1 risk factor is not necessary.

domized clinical trials have demonstrated the effectiveness of lipid-lowering therapy for preventing coronary artery disease.

Hypothyroidism

Many overweight or obese patients believe they must have a thyroid disorder. Secretion of thyroid hormone by the thyroid gland is regulated by thyroid stimulating hormone (TSH) produced by the pituitary gland. Most cases of hypothyroidism seen in clinical practice are the result of thyroid gland failure secondary to autoimmune destruction. These patients may show signs and symptoms, including fatigue, cold intolerance, constipation, hypertension, joint swelling, congestive heart failure, hyperlipidemia, or irregular menstrual periods in women. The single most useful screening laboratory test is a serum TSH level as measured by a sensitive second- or third-generation assay. The presence of thyroid peroxidase antibodies (TPO) or the older anti-microsomal or antithyroglobulin antibodies provides evidence of an autoimmune process directed at the thyroid gland, and should be considered as a follow-up test to an abnormal TSH level.

A patient with increased serum TSH level but a normal thyroid hormone concentration has a condition defined as subclinical hypothyroidism. It is reasonable to treat these individuals with thyroid hormone to a level that produces a normal TSH while looking for evidence of clinical improvement. Those patients found to have an increased TSH and a decreased T4 level have frank hypothyroidism. They probably will require life-long treatment

FIGURE 4.

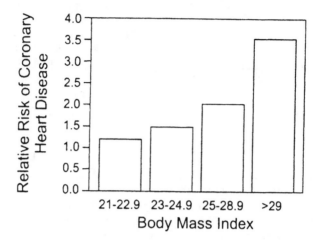

Body mass index and the risk of coronary disease.

with thyroid hormone replacement, although recent evidence suggests that 10–15% may eventually recover normal thyroid function.

In the absence of evidence of active coronary artery disease, thyroid hormone replacement can begin at a full replacement dose. The dose selected for a lean individual is roughly 1.5 to 1.6 micrograms/kilogram of body weight. While overweight or obese individuals require more thyroid hormone than lean individuals, this formula may overestimate replacement doses for these patients. Most obese individuals will require between 0.15–0.2 mg/day of levothyroxine. The half-life of thyroid hormone is roughly seven days. Allow a minimum of six weeks to elapse before checking another TSH level to assess the adequacy of therapy. The goal of treatment is to gradually increase the dose of thyroid hormone until the measured TSH value is between 1 and 2.5. If a repeat TSH is in the high normal range of 3 to 5, it is reasonable to try a slightly higher dose. If the TSH is below the normal range, the next lower dose should be prescribed.

Many overweight or obese patients have encountered information in the popular press or on the Internet that suggests this usual approach is inadequate for identifying and treating hypothyroidism. Some practitioners of alternative medicine advocate measuring basal body temperature and using USP thyroid, or T3 preparations at high doses. These writers suggest that many people are resistant to the usual pharmacologic preparations of thyroid hormone. Some weight-loss practitioners have advocated using high doses of thyroid hormone to promote weight loss. While it is biologically plausible that an individual could have isolated peripheral resistance to thyroid hormone, there have been no cases described in the scientific literature to

TABLE 5. Drugs Affecting Lipoprotein Metabolism*

Drug Class, Agents, and Daily Doses	Lipic/Lipoprotein Effects	Side Effects	Contraindications	Clinical Trial Results
HMG-CoA reductase inhibitors (statins)†	LDL ↓ 18%–55% HDL ↑ 5%–15% TG ↓ 7%–30%	Myopathy; increased liver enzymes	Absolute: active or chronic liver disease Relative: concomitant use of certain drugs§	Reduced major coronary events, CHD deaths, need for coronary procedures, stroke, and total mortality
Bile acid sequestrants‡	LDL ↓ 15%–30% HDL ↑ 3%–5% TG No change or increase	Gastrointestinal distress; constipation; decreased absorption of other drugs	Absolute: dysbetalipoproteinemia; TG > 400 mg/dL	Reduced major coronary events and CHD deaths
Nicotinic acid«	LDL ↓ 5%–25% HDL ↑ 15%–35% TG ↓ 20%–50%	Flushing; hyperglycemia; hyperuricemia (or gout); upper gastrointestinal distress; hepatotoxicity	Absolute: chronic liver disease; severe gout Relative: diabetes; hyperuricemia; peptic ulcer disease	Reduced major coronary events, and possibly total
Fibric acids¶	LDL ↓ 5%–20% (may be increased in patients with high TG) HDL ↑ 10%–20% TG ↓ 20%–50%	Dyspepsia; gallstones; myopathy; unexplained non-CHD deaths in WHO study	Absolute: severe renal disease; severe hepatic disease	Reduced major coronary events

*HMG-CoA indicates 3-hydroxy-3-methylglutaryl coenzyme A; LDL, low-density lipoprotein; HDL, high-density lipoprotein; TG, triglycerides; ↓, decrease; ↑, increase; and CHD, coronary heart disease.

†Lovastatin (20–80 mg), pravastatin (20–80 mg), simvastatin (20–40 mg) fluvastatin (20–80 mg), atorvastatin (10–80 mg), and cerivastatin (0.4–0.8 mg).

‡Cholestyramine (4–16 g), colestipol (5–20 g), and colesevelam (2.6–3.8 g).

§Cyclosporine, macrolide antibiotics, various antifungal agents, and cytochrome P-450 inhibitors (fibrates and niacin should be used with appropriate caution).

«Immediate-release (crystalline) nicotinic acid (1.5–3 g), extended-release nicotinic acid (1–2 g), and sustained-release nicotinic acid (1–2 g).

¶Gemfibrozil (600 mg twice daily), fenofibrate (200 mg), and clofibrate (1000 mg twice daily).

date. The use of USP thyroid or high doses of thyroid-hormone replacement puts the patient at risk for atrial arrhythmias, osteoporosis, and changes in mood or psychological functioning that could be detrimental for their health and functioning. For these reasons these practices are not within the scope of accepted medical practice, and should be considered to be outside the mainstream and associated with patient risk. Some specialists have advocated combining levothyroxine therapy with a daily dose of cytomel (T3). The problem with this practice is that the commercially available strength of cytomel may be too high for many patients. In general, this is not an accepted form of therapy at this time.

Cushing's Syndrome

Cushing's syndrome is a constellation of signs and symptoms caused by the overproduction of cortisol by the adrenal glands. It can be caused by a pituitary tumor secreting adrenocorticotropic hormone (ACTH), by ectopic production of ACTH, or by a tumor in one of the adrenal glands. The problem in evaluating an obese patient for Cushing's syndrome is that simple obesity itself can produce hypercortisolism that is difficult to distinguish from the hypercortisolism of Cushing's syndrome using the common screening tests. In addition, some of the findings generally associated with Cushing's syndrome can be seen in common forms of obesity. These include the presence of central obesity, a buffalo hump, supraclavicular fat pads, moonfacies, and the presence of diabetes or depression. Simple metabolic obesity can be associated with acne, hirsutism, and irregular menses in women. The more specific signs and symptoms of Cushing's syndrome include proximal muscle weakness, easy bruisability, osteoporosis, and wide purple striae (>1 cm). Patients with simple metabolic obesity are generally strong on neurologic testing. The presence of proximal muscle weakness warrants further evaluation, particularly if it has a recent onset or is progressive. While whitish or silvery striae are common in obese individuals, wide violaceous striae may be a clue to the presence of Cushing's syndrome. It is very uncommon for Cushing's syndrome to cause severe obesity. If a patient does not have some of these more specific signs of Cushing's syndrome, it is probably not worth pursuing the diagnosis given the risk of false-positive testing.

If further screening for Cushing's syndrome is warranted, there are two commonly used screening tests. The first is the overnight 1 mg dexamethasone suppression test. In this test, the patient takes a 1-mg oral dose of dexamethasone at 11 PM, then has blood drawn the following morning at 8 AM for a serum cortsiol level. A normal value is less than 5 ng/dl. The other screening test is the 24-hour urinary free cortisol. A value less than 100 is normal. Either test can be used, although many endocrinologists prefer the 24-hour urinary free cortisol because it tends to have fewer false-positive results. False-positive screening tests can be caused by medical illness, severe depression, alcohol abuse, or simple obesity. A normal screening test warrants reassurance of the patient, but if the test is abnormal, the patient

TABLE 6. A Guide to Selecting Treatment

Treatment	BMI Category				
	25–26.9	27–29.9	30–34.9	35–39.9	≥ 40
Diet, physical activity, and behavior therapy	With co-morbidities	With co-morbidities	+	+	+
Pharmacotherapy		With co-morbidities	+	+	+
Surgery				With co-morbidities	

- Prevention of weight gain with lifestyle therapy is indicated in any patient with a BMI ≥ 25 kg/m^2, even without co-morbidities, while weight loss is not necessarily recommended for those with a BMI of 25–29.9 kg/m^2 or a high waist circumference, unless they have two or more co-morbidities.

- Combined therapy with a low-calorie diet (LCD), increased physical activity, and behavior therapy provide the most successful intervention for weight loss and weight maintenance.

- Consider pharmacotherapy only if a patient has not lost 1 pound per week after 6 months of combined lifestyle therapy.

The + represents the use of indicated treatment regardless of co-morbidities.

should be referred to an endocrinologist for further evaluation. Several newer tests, such as dexamethasone suppression followed by corticotropic-releasing hormone (CRH) stimulation and salivary cortisol levels, have shown some utility in this difficult clinical situation.

■ Selecting and Suggesting a Treatment Modality

There are a number of treatment options available to help patients manage their weight. These include dietary modifications, increased physical activity, pharmacologic treatments, and surgery. These treatment approaches vary in both their effectiveness and risk. Diet and exercise have almost no risk and modest effectiveness. Drug therapy has more cost and risk yet adds effectiveness over diet and exercise used alone. Surgery has substantial risk and yet holds the promise of producing the most weight loss. The aggressiveness of the treatment approach should be tailored to match the health risks associated with the patient's weight (Table 6). Before selecting a treatment, it is important to collect information on the patient's usual diet and physical-activity habits, then determine his or her goals (chapter 5). Next asses patient readiness to change behaviors related to diet or physical activity (see chapter 6). Each patient will have unique feelings about how aggressively to treat his or her weight problem, however, it is helpful to have some guidelines as to which treatment might be optimal for which patient. The details of each of these treatment approaches will be discussed in subsequent chapters.

The issues discussed in this chapter are also covered in the "Practical Guide to the Identification, Evaluation and Treatment of Overweight and Obesity in

Adults" developed as part of the National Heart Lung and Blood Institute (NHLBI) of the National Institutes of Health's obesity education initiative in conjunction with the North American Association for the Study of Obesity. This excellent treatment guide can be obtained by contacting the NHLBI *Aim for a Healthy Weight* web page at www.nhlbi.nih.gov or by mail at:

National Heart Lung and Blood Institute
Education Programs Information Center
P.O. Box 30105
Bethesda, MD 20824-0105

References

1. The practical guide to the identification, evaluation and treatment of overweight and obesity in adults. NIH Publication Number 00-4084, Oct. 2000, at www.nhlbi.nih.gov.
2. Executive Summary of the Third Report of the National Cholesterol Education Program (NCEP) Expert Panel on Detection, Evaluation, and Treatment of High Blood Cholesterol in Adults (Adult Treatment Panel III). JAMA 285: 2486-97, 2001.
3. Position Statement: Screening for Diabetes. American Diabetes Association Clinical Practice Recommendations 2001. Diabetes Care 24 (Supplement 1), 2001.
4. Findling JW, Raff H: Newer diagnostic techniques and problems in Cushing's Disease. Endocrinol Metabol Clin North Am 28(1): 191-210, 1999.

Chapter 4

David Heber, MD, PhD, and Susan Bowerman, MS, RD

Body-Composition Analysis

With the incidence of overweight and obesity among adults in the United States at an all-time high and continuing to rise, the number of patients seeking advice for weight management is likely to parallel this trend. Most adults in primary care settings are overweight or obese, and two-thirds of patients with weight problems have obesity-related conditions.[1] Many primary care practitioners are reluctant to treat overweight and obese patients, citing lack of time, patient noncompliance, inadequate teaching materials, lack of counseling training, inadequate reimbursement, and low physician confidence as barriers to treatment.[2-8] Among those who do address dietary issues with their patients, the time spent discussing weight management has been reported to be 5 minutes or less.[2] Even though time is a concern, appropriate assessment is critical in counseling and management of patients who are overweight or obese.

■ Patient Assessment

There has been increasing attention paid to the use of the body mass index (BMI) as the "fifth vital sign" in assessing the patient. The BMI (weight (kg)/height (meters)^2) approximates total body fat based on height and weight, and can be useful for a quick assessment in the majority of cases; further, an individual's risk for type 2 diabetes, hypertension, and cardiovascular disease are based on BMI (see chapter 3). Waist circumference is used as an additional assessment of risk because it is an independent measure in those with central obesity, and because waist circumference loses its predictive power in determining risk for co-morbid conditions once the BMI reaches 35 or greater.

While BMI gives a general idea of the degree of obesity (or excess fat) in populations, in certain groups such as the elderly or very muscular athletes, BMI will give an inaccurate indication of obesity due to significant variations in lean body mass. Additionally, obese subjects can be divided into three categories: (1) sarcopenic obese, characterized by excess body fat and reduced lean body mass; (2) normal obese with excess body fat and proportionate lean body mass; and (3) hypermuscular obese, with increased body fat and increased lean body mass.

Increased lean mass as well as fat mass is seen in many obese individuals. Drenick, using total body potassium, found increased lean tissue in obese adults.[9] Webster et al. measured the body composition of 104 obese and normal weight women by densitometry and reported that the excess body weight of the obese over non-obese women consisted of 22 to 30% lean and 70 to 78% fat tissue.[10] Forbes and Welle[11] examined data on lean body mass in obese subjects collected in their laboratory or published in the literature. Their own data demonstrated that 75% of the obese population had a lean-to-height ratio that exceeded 1 standard deviation (SD) and that more than half exceeded 2 SD. A review of the literature supported these observations and determined that the lean body mass could account for approximately 29% of excess weight in obese patients. A proportionate increase of lean body mass of approximately 25% is considered normal.

Deviations both above and below this amount of lean mass are observed on clinical grounds based on various etiologies. Sarcopenic obesity can result from chronic use of corticosteroids, prolonged inactivity or bed rest, hypogonadism, hypopituitarism, neuromuscular diseases, menopause and age-related hypogonadism, and genetic influences. Hypermuscular obesity can result from childhood onset severe obesity, use of anabolic androgens, hyperandrogenism in females, athletics (e.g., football, wrestling, weightlifting), and genetic influences.

In those overweight individuals with higher than average lean body mass, body-composition analysis can be used to calculate a more appropriate target weight than would be predicted from ideal body weight tables. Hypermuscular obese patients are often relieved to learn that their target weights are higher than what would be predicted from standard reference tools for appropriate weight for height. In those obese subjects with reduced lean body mass, a program of aerobic and heavy resistance training can be initiated to provide for an increase in lean body mass and therefore energy expenditure.

Lean body mass predicts energy expenditure, and from this, the rate of weight loss on a given calorie-restricted diet can be predicted.[12] In both markedly obese individuals and individuals with decreased lean body mass, there is linear relationship of lean body mass to energy expenditure such that each pound of lean body mass burns approximately 13.8 kilocalories per day. This represents approximately 90% of total energy expenditure in a sedentary obese individual and can provide a good clinical estimate of maintenance calories in these patients.

In addition, lean body mass can be used to estimate dietary protein needs. Most individuals need between 0.5–1.0 grams of dietary protein per pound of lean body mass per day, depending upon their level of activity and personal goals. Individuals who are attempting to build muscle would do well to aim closer to the 1.0 gram/pound range.

There are several methods of body-composition analysis, including anthropometry (the use of calipers for skinfold measurements), near-infrared interactance (NIA), hydrostatic weighing, air displacement, dual energy x-ray absorptiometry (DEXA), and bioelectrical impedance (BIA).

Anthropometry

Using hand-held calipers that exert a standard pressure, the skinfold thickness is measured at various body locations (3–7 test sites are common). A calculation is then used to derive a body fat percentage based on the sum of the measurements. The caliper method is based upon the assumption that the thickness of the subcutaneous fat reflects a constant proportion of the total body fat and that the sites selected for measurement represent the average thickness of the subcutaneous fat.

Skinfold measurements are made by grasping the skin and underlying tissue, shaking it to exclude any muscle, and pinching it between the jaws of the calipers. Duplicate readings are often made at each site to improve the accuracy and reproducibility of the measurements. Generally speaking, skinfold measurements are easy, inexpensive, and portable. However, results can be very subjective as precision ultimately depends on the skill of the person making the measurement and the site measured. The quality of the calipers is also a factor; they should be accurately calibrated and have a constant specified pressure. Inexpensive models sold for the home use are usually less accurate than those used by an accredited caliper technician. The more obese the subject, the more difficult it is to "pinch" the skinfold correctly, requiring even more skill to obtain an accurate measurement.

Near-Infrared Interactance

In this method, a fiber optic probe is connected to a digital analyzer that indirectly measures the tissue composition (fat and water) at various sites on the body. This method is based on studies that show optical densities are linearly related to subcutaneous and total body fat. The biceps is the most often used single site for estimating body fat using the NIR method. The NIR light penetrates the tissues and is reflected off the bone back to the detector. The NIR data is entered into a prediction equation with the person's height, weight, frame size, and level of activity to estimate the percent body fat.

This method has become popular outside of the laboratory because it is simple, fast, noninvasive, and relatively inexpensive. However, the amount of pressure applied to the fiberoptic probe during measurement may affect the values of optical densities, and skin color and hydration level may be potential sources of error. To date, studies conducted with this method have produced mixed results: a high degree of error has occurred with very lean and very obese people, and the validity of a single-site measurement at the biceps is questionable. Much more research is needed to substantiate the validity, accuracy, and applicability of this method, and it is therefore not recommended.

Hydrostatic Weighing

Hydrostatic weighing measures whole-body density by determining body volume. There is a variety of equipment available to do underwater weighing ranging in sophistication from the standard stainless steel tank with a chair or cot mounted on underwater scales to a chair and scale suspended from a diving board over a pool or hot tub.

The individual is first weighed outside the tank, then immersed totally in water and weighed again. Since bone and muscle are more dense and fat is less dense than water, an individual with more bone and muscle will weigh more in water and therefore have a higher body density and lower percentage of body fat than an individual who has a higher proportion of body fat. The volume of the body is calculated and the individual's body density is determined using standard formulas. Body fat percentage is then calculated from body density using standard equations.

The underlying assumption with this method is that densities of fat mass and fat-free mass are constant. However, underwater weighing may not be the appropriate gold standard for everyone. For example, athletes tend to have denser bones and muscles than non-athletes, which may lead to an underestimation of body fat percentage. At the same time, the body fat of elderly patients suffering from osteoporosis may be overestimated. To date, specific equations have not been developed to accommodate these different population groups.

Another important consideration in this method is residual lung volume, which can be estimated or measured, but a direct measure is desirable and it should be taken in the tank whenever possible.

Air Displacement

Based on the same principle as underwater weighing, the BOD POD is a fiberglass plethysmograph that measures body volume by changes in pressure in a closed chamber. The system uses computerized sensors to measure how much air is displaced while a person sits within the chamber. It uses a calculation to determine body density, then estimates body fat. The system is safe, relatively quick, results are easily replicated, and the chamber can accommodate a wide range of body shapes and sizes. However, the equipment is very expensive and limited in availability. Another drawback to this method is that subjects need to be clothed in very tight-fitting attire, including a tight-fitting swim cap, for accurate measurement. Since the equipment is measuring air displacement, uncovered scalp hair and loose clothing can underestimate body fat by more than two percent and five percent, respectively.[13,14]

Dual Energy X-ray Absorptiometry (DEXA)

The use of DEXA for body composition analysis is based on a three-compartment model that divides the body into total body mineral, fat-free lean mass, and fat tissue mass. DEXA uses a whole body scanner which has two low-dose x-rays at different sources that read bone and soft tissue mass simultaneously. The sources are mounted beneath a table with a detector overhead. The scanner passes across the individual's reclining body and data is collected at 0.5-cm intervals. The full scan takes between 10 and 20 minutes. It is safe and noninvasive, although the individual must lie still throughout the procedure.

DEXA is becoming regarded as the new "gold standard" in body composition analysis because it provides a higher degree of precision in only one measurement, and can also show the distribution of fat tissue throughout the body. It is very reliable and the results reproducible. However, the equipment is not widely available, although it is moving more from the laboratory into clinical settings. In evaluating fat mass by DEXA as compared to bioelectrical impedance or skinfold thickness, body fat is underestimated by the other methods as compared to DEXA, with better precision obtained by the DEXA.[15] In nonobese patients, skinfold thickness or bioelectrical impedance is appropriate for routine monitoring, but DEXA may be the method of choice in obese patient monitoring, since reproducibility gains special importance.

Bioelectrical Impedance (BIA)

Bioelectrical impedance analysis is a relatively quick, simple, and fairly accurate way to determine body composition. For the analysis, the patient only needs to remove the shoe and sock on one foot. Gel electrodes are placed on the hands and feet, and a very mild electrical current is sent through the body. Muscle, because it contains water and electrolytes, will conduct the current; fat tissue acts as an insulator and resists the current. The differences in conduction between the two tissues provide the machine with a measure of electrical impedance, which is then applied to a mathematical formula to calculate lean body mass. The entire procedure takes only a few minutes, and the instrument provides information on fat mass in pounds and percentage of total body weight, lean body mass in pounds and percent, basal metabolic rate based on lean body mass, and target weight.

During the first week of caloric restriction, there is a loss of body weight in excess of the loss of lean and fat tissue due to a water diuresis. If patients are measured at their first visit and then frequently thereafter, it is possible to find that patients are apparently gaining fat as they lose weight using bioelectrical impedance. Since lean body mass is assessed based on both body water and muscle, the loss of water leads to an apparent decrease in lean body mass, which in most cases exceeds the loss of fat in the first week of dieting, leading to a seeming increase in percent body fat.[16] The bioelectrical impedance measurement is most useful at the first visit for assessing type of obesity, and not useful for multiple serial determinations.

A second potential problem is overemphasis on the quantitative accuracy of body fat estimation. Small changes cannot be measured using this device, and it is important to stress this fact to patients. The changes observed in percent fat often do not impress patients as much as the ratio of the absolute change in fat mass in pounds compared to changes in lean mass.

■ Summary

It is important for doctors and other health care providers to understand the value of body-composition analysis and the individualized approaches to diet that take into consideration muscle mass and protein requirements. Since many patients have unrealistic expectations about weight loss, body composition assessment can play a useful role in establishing a patient's target weight. Studies have shown the great impact of personalized knowledge of cholesterol or blood pressure on lifestyle changes. Personalized information on target weight and resting metabolic rate could have a similar beneficial impact on lifestyle changes required for effective weight management.

References

1. Logue E, Sutton K, Jarjoura D, Smucker W: Obesity management in primary care: assessment of readiness to change among 284 family practice patients. J Am Board Fam Pract 13:164-71, 2000.
2. Kushner RF: Barriers to providing nutrition counseling by physicians: a survey of primary care practitioners. Prev Med 24:546-52, 1995.
3. Hiddink Gj, Hautvast JG, van Woerkum CM, Fieren CJ, van't Hof MA: Nutrition guidance by primary-care physicians: perceived barriers and low involvement. Eur J Clin Nutr 49:842-51, 1995.
4. Pratt CA, Nosiri UI, Pratt CB: Michigan physicians' perceptions of their role in managing obesity. Percept Mot Skills 84:848-50, 1997.
5. Truswell AS: Family physicians and patients: is effective nutrition interaction possible? Am J Clin Nut 71:6-12, 2000.
6. Helman A: Nutrition and general practice: an Australian perspective. Am J Clin Nutr 65:1939S-42, 1997.
7. Harris JE, Hamaday V, Mochan E: Osteopathic family physicians' attitudes, knowledge and self-reported practices regarding obesity. J Am Osteopath Assoc 99:358-365, 1999.
8. Kenner MM, Taylor ML, Dunn PC, Gruchow HW, Kolasa K: Primary care providers need a variety of nutrition and wellness patient education materials. J Am Diet Assoc 99:4662-466, 1999.
9. Drenick EJ, Blahd WH, Singer FR, et al: Body potassium content in obese subjects and postassium depletion during prolonged fasting. Am J Clin Nutr 18:278-285, 1966.
10. Webster JD, Hesp R, Garrow JS: The composition of excess weight in obese women estimated by body density, total body water, and total body potassium. Human Nutrition:
11. Forbes GB, Welle SL: Lean body mass in obesity. Int J Obesity 7:99-107, 1983.
12. Yang M-U: Body composition and resting metabolic rate in obesity. In: Obesity and Weight Control (Frankle RT and Yang M-U, eds.) Aspen Publishers, Rockville, 1988, pp 71-96.
13. Higgins, PG, Fields DA, Hunter GR, Gower BA: Effect of scalp and facial hair on air displacement plethysmography estimates of percentage of body fat. Obes Res May;9(5):326-30, 2001.
14. Fields DA, Hunter GR, Goran MI: Validation of the BOD POD with hydrostatic weighing: influence of body clothing. Int J Obes Relat Metab Disord 24(2):200-5, 2000.
15. Erselcan T, Candan F, Saruhan S, Ayca T: Comparison of body composition analysis methods in clinical routine. Ann Nutr Metab 44 (5-6):243-8, 2000.
16. Gray DS: Changes in bioelectrical impedance during fasting. Am J Clin Nutr 48:1184-1187, 1998.

Chapter 5

Gary D. Foster, Ph.D.

Goals and Strategies to Improve Behavior-Change Effectiveness

Independent of the treatment modality selected (balanced deficit diet, pharmacotherapy, or surgery), the endpoint of obesity treatment is to help patients eat less and move more. This chapter reviews some practical aspects of helping patients change their eating and activity patterns, including talking empathically with patients about weight control, improving adherence to eating and activity plans, and helping patients accept weight losses that are less than their ideal.

■ Talking with Patients about Weight Control

No matter what type of obesity treatment is ultimately recommended, effective and compassionate treatment of obese patients requires an understanding of the cultural context in which treatment occurs. As Stunkard and Sobal have suggested, disparagement of obese individuals is the last socially acceptable form of prejudice. It is not surprising, therefore, that health care providers seem to share society's negative view of the overweight. In one study, 63% of family practice physicians attributed obesity to a lack of willpower, and more than a third described their obese patients as "lazy." Such characterizations are likely to lead to discriminatory behaviors. There are numerous clinical anecdotes about how obese patients have been treated disrespectfully in the medical setting.

■ Toward More Empathic Encounters

It can be argued that overweight patients are "just too sensitive," and their perceptions about medical visits reflect their own frustration with their weight rather than any systemic bias by health care professionals. Even if patients' bad experiences are partly due to inaccurate perceptions, such experiences need to be remedied. These inaccurate perceptions lead to interactions that, at best, provide medical care at the expense of a patient's self-esteem or, at worst, prevent obese patients from seeking health care altogether. The following recommendations, based on the available research as well as clinical experience, seek to put obese patients at ease in the medical setting and promote competent, compassionate care.

Assume that obese individuals know they are overweight. If they have not heard it from a health care professional, they have probably been told by friends, family, or even strangers. Simple phrases such as, "What do you think about your weight?" will allow you to assess the patient's interest and/or motivation for weight control in a non-judgmental fashion. They also allow you to hear the patient's perspective *before* making any recommendations for weight loss or describing the ill effects of excess weight.

Listen carefully to the patient's presenting problem, independent of weight. Few patients consider weight to be their primary problem. As Stunkard points out, patients define the presenting problem. If weight is a precipitating condition, focus on the factors that affect the presenting problem and weight. For example, it is not likely to be useful to tell an obese patient with dyslipidemia to lose weight. Encouraging the same patient to decrease their intake of saturated fat and make small changes in activity, however, will likely influence weight and lipids. Such advice is better received by patients who are often told to lose weight in response to many medical problems.

Provide the same care to obese patients as to nonobese patients. Lean individuals with hypertension or type-2 diabetes are encouraged to watch their diets but are also provided appropriate medication for their conditions. Too often, obese patients are told to lose weight, and appropriate pharmacologic care may not be provided in a timely manner.

Create a User-Friendly Office

Just as airline seats are frequently too small for significantly obese patients, so are the equipment and furnishings found in many medical practices. Attention to the following details facilitates an environment that is receptive to obese patients.

Have a scale that can weigh all patients. Getting weighed is among the most unpleasant experiences for an obese patient in the medical setting; it becomes tortuous and humiliating if a patient weighs more than the scale can accommodate.

Have gowns available that fit larger patients. Many obese patients report the experience of waiting for a physician examination in a gown that barely covers them.

Use larger blood pressure cuffs when appropriate. Office staff should know when to use larger cuffs with patients. Inappropriate cuff sizes will lead to inaccurate measurements and treatment recommendations.

Provide some armless chairs in your waiting room. Obese patients should not be made to feel uncomfortable in chairs made for lean persons. Other practical suggestions for creating an office environment that is friendly for obese patients are discussed in chapter 2.

Improving Adherence

The principles and practices of the behavioral treatment of obesity have been reviewed in detail elsewhere. Some helpful references are included at the end of this chapter. However, several straightforward guidelines can help patients improve their adherence to the behaviors necessary for effective weight control. Keeping some of the focus on specific behavior change goals as opposed to target weight loss goals will improve adherence and success.

Establish a specific plan (WHAT). Help patients select a specific plan (limit eating to 300 kcal between 7:00-10:00 PM or walk three times for twenty minutes after dinner on Monday, Wednesday, and Friday) rather than a general platitude (eat less at night or exercise more). The more specific the goal, the better.

Identify facilitators and barriers to success (HOW). Help patients think through what steps will be necessary to achieve their goal (purchasing alternative foods for evening consumption or having a spouse help with household duties after dinner).

Follow-up at the next visit. Have the patient make a written record of the plan and key steps in its implementation. In addition, make a brief note in the chart documenting the specific plan. At the next visit, review the patient's progress with the plan. If successful, what strategies did the patient use to achieve the goal? If unsuccessful, what things got in the way, and how can they be removed in the future? Patients benefit more from examining **how** behavior changed or did not change rather than focusing on **why** things did not go as planned.

Avoid criticizing patients. Weight control is tough work and patients need to know that you will not give up on them. Help patients identify problem areas and take responsibility for addressing them. Criticizing patients or questioning their motivation does little for improving adherence and has adverse effects on the patient-physician relationship.

■ Unrealistic Expectations

One of the greatest challenges in the clinical management of obese patients is the significant disparity between actual and expected weight losses. While professionals generally accept a 10% weight loss as successful (based on the associated improvements in co-morbidities), patients typically seek weight losses that approximate 30% reductions in body weight. Several recommendations may help patients accept more modest weight loss outcomes as successful.

Be clear about what weight loss does and does not. Weight loss will make you healthier, but it does not guarantee a better job, a happier marriage, or other things that many patients seek through weight loss. Discussing (before treatment) what else patients expect to change besides weight will help identify any unrealistic expectations or magical thinking regarding weight loss.

Focus on non-weight outcomes. Focus on the many non-weight changes such as improvements in serum lipids, blood pressure, and glycemic control. In addition, prompt patients to assess changes in their quality of life such as increased energy, being able to keep up with children or grandchildren, and climbing stairs without shortness of breath.

Discuss biological limits. In short, acknowledge what patients already know: not everyone who eats the same and exercises the same weighs the same. Weight is not infinitely malleable, and there are likely biological boundaries that set limits for weight loss. Help patients focus on behavioral changes that improve health and worry less about the ultimate number of pounds lost. Patients will need your help to counter the cultural myth that "you can weigh whatever you want."

Be empathic about dissatisfaction with weight and/or shape. It is reassuring for patients to hear from their physicians things like, "Weight control is really tough work, isn't it?" or, "It must be frustrating to have worked so hard and still be unhappy because you haven't lost as much weight as you wanted." Such phrases let patients know that the physician understands their difficulties and will not be judgmental.

Encourage a weight-independent self-esteem. Physicians can provide a great service to obese patients by reminding them that their worth is not measured on the scale. Patients should be encouraged to take themselves, their health, and their weight seriously rather than attempting to lose weight so they can like themselves. Reaffirming the patient's self-worth, independent of body weight, is perhaps one of the most powerful interventions a physician can provide an obese patient.

Suggested Readings

Physician Resources

Foster GD and Johnson C: Facilitating health and self-dsteem among obese patients. Prim Psychiatr 5:89-95, 1998.

Foster GD, Wadden TA, Vogt RA, Brewer G: What is a reasonable weight loss? Patients' expectations and evaluations of obesity treatment outcomes. J Consulting and Clin Psychol 65: 79-85, 1997.

Stunkard AJ: Talking with patients. In Stunkard AJ and Wadden TA (eds): Obesity: Theory and Therapy. 2nd ed. New York, Raven Press; 1993, pp. 355-363.

Stunkard AJ, Sobal J: Psychosocial consequences of obesity. In Brownell KD and Fairburn CG (eds): Eating Disorders and Obesity: A Comprehensive Handbook. New York, Guilford Press; 1995, pp. 417-421.

Wadden TA, Foster GD: Behavioral treatment of obesity. In Jensen M (ed): Medical Clinics of North America. 2000, 84:2, 441-61.

Wadden TA, Wingate BJ: Compassionate treatment of the obese individual. In Brownell KD and Fairburn CG (eds), Eating Disorders and Obesity: A Comprehensive Handbook. New York, Guilford Press; 1995, pp. 564-71.

Patient Resources

Brownell KD: The Learn Program for Weight Management 2000. Dallas, American Health, 2000.

Cash TF: The Body Image Workbook. Oakland, CA, New Harbinger Publications, 1997.

Johnson CA: Self-Esteem Comes in All Sizes. Carlsbad CA, Gurze Books, 2001.

Chapter 6

Daniel H. Bessesen, MD

Applying Stages of Change Theory to Office-based Counseling

The ten-minute office visit is a difficult format for meaningful behavioral counseling. Most clinical care providers experience some frustration when dealing with overweight and obese patients in an office setting. Some of this frustration comes from the limitations of time, but some comes from a change in the usual relationships between the care provider, the patient, and their disease (Figure 1). In any clinic encounter there are important interactions between these three players. For many health care problems encountered in the clinic, the primary interaction is between the care provider and the disease: the care provider evaluates the nature of the disease and prescribes treatment. The patient is asking for advice and usually follows clinician suggestions. In these situations the care provider is able to "manage" the disease for the patient (Figure 2). Diseases such as urinary tract infections, pneumonia, or acute chest pain require immediate attention from the care provider. In these settings the care provider, acting as the "manager," is in control, responsible, in charge of decision-making, and accountable for the outcome.

However, when dealing with health-related behaviors such as eating and physical activity, the care provider is placed in a subtly different role. In these interactions the care provider may reflexively assume the role of the manager, diagnosing the condition and prescribing treatment. However, in these situations the *patient* is the person in control, responsible, and experiencing the consequences of the behavior.

■ The Role of the Care Provider

In these situations a more realistic role for the clinician is "consultant" or even "coach" (Figure 3). A good consultant recognizes that he or she is not the decision-maker, not in control, and not ultimately responsible for the outcome. A good consultant is an expert and a good listener who believes that the patient has good reason for doing whatever he or she is currently doing, although the decisions may also have adverse consequences. The first step in consulting is understanding the motives for the patient's actions. The next step is working with the patient to appreciate the implications of behaviors on health, and moving that behavior in a direction that would promote health.

FIGURE 1.

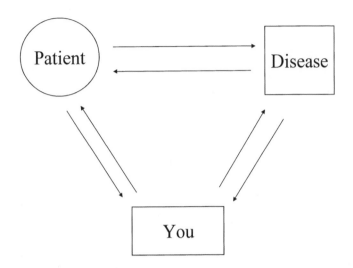

■ Stages of Change Theory

The stages of change theory developed by Prochaska and DiClemente were initially applied to counseling for cigarette smoking.[1] However, change theory can provide a useful framework for a care provider counseling a patient about his or her eating and physical activity habits. Prochaska and DiClemente hypothesized that individuals go through the following predictable stages as they change from established behaviors to new behaviors.[2]

Precontemplative
Contemplative
Planning
Action
Maintenance
Relapse

Moving a patient from inaction to action in one office visit is probably an unrealistic goal and may frustrate the care provider. A more productive approach is to determine the patient's motivation for behavior change and target counseling efforts at incrementally moving to the next stage in the process. Determining what stage the patient is in and focusing the clinic visit on that stage allows more efficient use of time and increases the chance of success.

To determine the stage of the patient, the clinician needs to examine the current behaviors and how the patient feels about these behaviors. If the clinician is interested in altering diet, then start with a 1–3 day diet recall history (see chapter 7 on taking a dietary history). If the clinician wants to discuss physical activity, start by asking the patient about planned and

FIGURE 2.

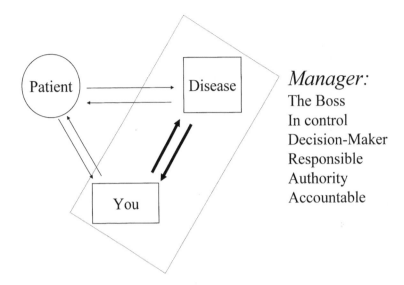

Manager:
The Boss
In control
Decision-Maker
Responsible
Authority
Accountable

unplanned physical activity over the last 2 weeks (see chapter 12 on taking a physical activity history). Then the care provider can explore whether the patient is interested in discussing behavior change strategies. Having a "script" of important discussion points for each stage of change can make the clinic encounter less stressful and more productive for the care provider.

Precontemplative

If the patient reacts to questions about the nature of their diet with a look of confusion, having only a vague recollection of what was eaten the previous day, he or she is probably in a precontemplative stage. Time could be spent exploring whether the individual thinks that diet has any relationship with current state of health. If not, this patient is in the precontemplative state.

The main task of the clinician counseling an individual in the precontemplative stage is to give a clear statement, in a supportive manner, that diet choices have health consequences, and that help is available should he or she choose to change dietary habits. Many clinicians use this approach in counseling patients to stop smoking. In that situation, the clinician makes a clear non-judgmental statement that smoking has adverse health consequences and that there would likely be health benefits if the individual stopped, and then offers assistance should the patient choose to stop. A similar approach can be used for the overweight patient who has not yet considered changing their diet.

Contemplative

The contemplative individual has already identified that diet may have adverse health consequences, but he or she sees many barriers to changing

FIGURE 3.

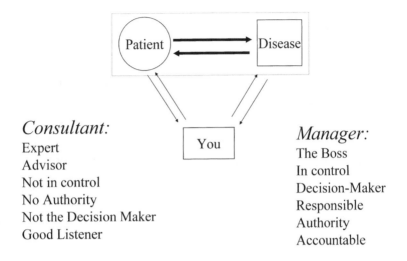

Consultant:
Expert
Advisor
Not in control
No Authority
Not the Decision Maker
Good Listener

Manager:
The Boss
In control
Decision-Maker
Responsible
Authority
Accountable

behavior. At this stage, providing detailed instructions of what to eat may not be appropriate, because these individuals need help problem-solving around barriers to behavior change. Who does the food purchasing in the house? Are meals eaten outside the home? Are there unrealistic expectations of how dramatic diet change needs to be? Exploring the answers to these questions may help this kind of an individual move toward actual planning for a change in dietary habits.

Planning and Action

A person in this stage has already identified adverse health effects of a poor diet, and he or she is ready to try changing it. The primary task for the care provider in this type of encounter is to assist the individual in developing a clear plan for the task. Helping the person identify potential problems and developing strategies for overcoming them may improve the chances of success. Small achievable steps are important (see chapter 7 on dietary counseling). Keep a positive environment and identify and encourage any success.

Some individuals at this stage already have strong ideas for proceeding. The patient might say, "I am going on that Atkins Diet. That guy really knows what he is talking about! The suggestions that you have always made about low fat diets have never worked for me." The care provider should avoid an initial reaction to argue with the wisdom of the decision. Instead consider that the patient has already overcome many hurdles, and it may be important to harness the energy and support his or her decision. An opportunity now exists to provide objective information on the health effects of his or her choices (see chapter 10 on fad diets).

Maintenance

Individuals in the maintenance phase have already examined behaviors, identified new options, and established new patterns of eating. However, experience shows that many people who have changed their diet may have difficulty sustaining that behavior change. The counseling task during a clinic visit with a patient at this stage is to support the behavior change with positive encouragement, to emphasize the need for long-term maintenance of the new behaviors, and to look for potential problems that may lie ahead. Holidays or celebrations may produce dietary indiscretion, and "diet fatigue" or boredom with an overly restrictive regimen are common challenges to diet maintenance. Developing strategies for these scenarios may give the patient confidence that he or she can maintain long-term success with the chosen dietary program.

Relapse

Most people who attempt weight loss using behavioral strategies try and fail several times before ultimately succeeding (see chapter 17 on the National Weight Control Registry). Most clinicians experience this in smoking cessation as well. It is important to appreciate that relapse is a common if not universal part of behavior change. The care provider should be able to identify the person in relapse and offer a well-thought-out approach to a person in this stage. An individual in relapse may say, "I have tried diets before. They never work for me. I will never be able to change my diet," exhibiting feeling of hopelessness.

A strategy for a relapse visit might begin by letting the patient know how common this is, that it is a natural and even expected part of dieting. The biologic nature of obesity can be discussed. The difficulties inherent in changing behavior can be acknowledged. The care provider can probe for previous dieting efforts and give positive feedback on successful efforts. Many of these patients actually have succeeded in losing weight before. They should be congratulated on those previous efforts, and reasons why previous behavior changes were not sustained can be explored. Were there unrealistic expectations of weight loss? Did a particular life event trigger a relapse? Could they now envision alternative approaches that build on those previous experiences? Moving the individual in relapse back to a pre-contemplative state might be a highly successful outcome of the office visit. Alternatively, identifying that this may not be the right time to embark on another attempt at behavior change may be another positive outcome. Supporting the patient's self-esteem in this setting is critical. Let them know that accepting their weight where it is may be the best option for now. Helping an individual like this separate personal identity and worth from body weight and appearance is an important intervention.

■ Counseling about Behavior Change

In counseling individuals about behavior change, have patients formally look at their own perceptions about existing and future behaviors. A 2×2 table,

FIGURE 4.

	Pros	Cons
Old Behavior	1._____ 2._____ 3._____ 4._____ 5._____	1._____ 2._____ 3._____ 4._____ 5._____
New Behavior	1._____ 2._____ 3._____ 4._____ 5._____	1._____ 2._____ 3._____ 4._____ 5._____

a list of pros and cons for old behaviors and new behaviors (Figure 4) is some-times useful. An individual stuck in current behaviors is indicating that the pros of that behavior outweigh the pros of future behavior. They see the negatives of current behaviors as outweighed by the negatives of the new behavior. Having the patient explicitly record the good and bad aspects of current and future behaviors may help them objectively decide between the two.

A patient may continue a current diet out of lifestyle considerations—it is convenient and it tastes good (pros). He or she may also see that the current diet causes weight gain and has other adverse health affects (cons). The patient understands that a behavior change to a more healthy diet is positive and that it may improve health, but he or she may be unsure of the magni-tude of those benefits. A healthier diet may cost more, not taste as good, and leave him or her feeling hungry much of the time. If the benefits of the new behavior outweigh the benefits of the current behavior (and similarly that the disadvantages of the current behavior outweigh the disadvantage of the new behavior), then behavior change will follow naturally (Figure 5). Having the patient commit these ideas to paper outlines for the care provider how best to discuss the issues involved and promote a change in behavior.

■ Summary

The ten-minute office visit is a difficult format for counseling patients about changing diet and physical activity patterns. Both the health care provider and the overweight patient should keep expectations realistic. Fif-teen years ago many clinicians did not discuss smoking cessation with

FIGURE 5.

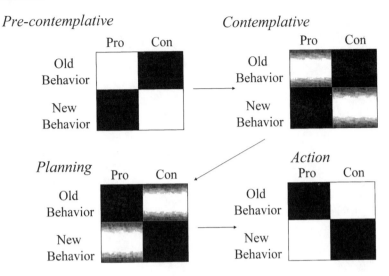

patients because there seemed little hope for success. Today, care providers realize that a little time spent encouraging behavior change may, over time, form a foundation on which people do change behaviors. This same rationale can be used with overweight and obese patients. The role of the clinician in an encounter with an overweight or obese patient is to support that individual as they strive for health-related behaviors that meet the specific needs of their life.

References

1. Prochazka, JO DiClemente CC, et al. Standardized, individualized, interactive, and personalized self-help programs for smoking cessation. Health Psychol 12:399-405, 1993.
2. Velicer, WF, Hughes SL, et al. An empirical typology of subjects within stage of change. Addict Behav 20:299-320, 1995.

Chapter 7

Dawn Jackson, RD, Amy Baltes, RD, and Robert Kushner, MD

Diets

■ General Principles

The typical American diet has increased from 1,854 calories in 1978 to 2,002 calories in 1996. Over the past 30 years, there have been increases in consumption of foods like cheese, added fats (salad dressings and cooking oils), refined grains (pasta, chips, and ready-to-eat cereals), and record increases in the use of caloric sweeteners (approximately 53 added teaspoonfuls per person per day). Also noteworthy, the food budget spent away from home/dining out has increased from 25% in 1970 to 40% in the late nineties.[1] The typical American diet is responsible in large part for the fact that 3 out of 5 people coming into a physician's office are overweight.

Recommendations for Americans have been made by many top health organizations such as the American Heart Association, American Cancer Society, American Dietetic Association, and the National Institutes of Health. These organizations have come to a consensus on dietary recommendations called the "Unified Diet."[2] These dietary guidelines include: 55–60% carbohydrate, 15–20% protein, and <30% fat (less than 10% saturated, up to 15% monounsaturated, up to 10% polyunsaturated).

The following are practical recommendations to help patients achieve dietary goals. When prescribing a diet, it is important to remember the role of nutrition in total health, not just weight loss:

1. Eat at least 5–7 servings of fruits and vegetables per day
2. Eat 25–30 grams of fiber per day (from fruits/vegetables, whole grain breads, cereals, pastas, crackers, and beans)
3. Choose whole grains over refined, processed carbohydrates
4. Drink at least 64 ounces of water each day
5. Eat at least 2 servings of low-fat dairy per day
6. Choose more low-fat proteins like skinless chicken, turkey, and soy products while choosing leaner cuts of beef and pork
7. Eat fish at least two times per week
8. Limit sodium intake to 2,400 mg per day

■ Weight-loss Diets

A key element of a weight loss diet is the use of moderate calorie reductions to achieve a slow and progressive weight loss. A diet with a goal of weight loss needs to have a 500 to 1,000 kcal/day deficit to achieve a 1–2 pound weight loss per week. In January 2001, the USDA white papers stated, "In the absence of physical activity, a diet that contains about 1,400–1,500 calories per day, regardless of macronutrient composition, results in weight loss."[3] The translation of this information is, controlling *calories* is the bottom line to a weight loss diet.

■ Producing a Calorie Deficit

Calories can be reduced by changing food **choices** and changing food **portions**. Making small, continuous, incremental improvements in behaviors is an effective way to produce a calorie deficit and improve the overall quality of a diet. This principle helps patients incorporate foods they enjoy without feeling a total sense of deprivation. Food is much more to people than just nourishment. It is comfort, stress relief, socialization, and a cure for boredom, frustration, and depression. Going slow is the best approach, and the first step to counseling a patient on weight loss and small sustainable changes in food choices and/or food portions is to find out what they are currently eating.

■ Monitoring Patient Eating

Two commonly used techniques to understand patients' eating patterns/habits are a typical day recall and food journals. A typical day recall is best used during a brief office visit. If more long-term counseling is desired, a food journal can be given to the patient for completion for the next appointment.

A typical day recall is obtained by asking the question, "Please take me through your typical diet, beginning when you wake up in the morning and continuing into the evening." When using a typical day recall, prompt the patient for information like timing and location of eating/snacking, specific food choices and portions, beverages consumed/water intake, and hunger levels.

Asking the patient to keep a food journal will offer insight into behaviors and environmental influences contributing to weight gain. Lifestyle patterns can more easily be detected with daily food journals than with a basic typical day recall. Additionally, patients who record their daily intake in food journals tend to be more conscientious about food choices and portions than their counterparts not keeping a journal.

■ Suggestions for Altering Pattern and Behavior

The following table includes habits patients are likely to report and brief therapeutic suggestions.

Common findings	Suggested therapeutic strategies
Nighttime eating	Make sure to not skip meals during the day. Try to substitute other behaviors in place of eating in the evening like taking a bath, listening to music, writing a letter to a friend, etc.
Binge eating	Make sure to not skip meals during the day. Consciously avoid situations and places that trigger binge behavior.

	*Note: Binge eating disorder, BED, is a psychological condition that may need additional attention.
Trigger foods	Keep trigger foods out of sight and plan to eat them only in "safe" conditions where no bingeing can occur.
Portions too large	Become familiar with recommended portion sizes. Pre-portion foods on plate and do not opt for second servings. Share entrées when eating out.
Emotional eating (stress, boredom, etc.)	Become aware of when emotional eating occurs and try to substitute other activities like deep breathing, going for a walk, or talking to a friend.
Too many snacks	Pre-plan healthy snacks like yogurt and high fiber cereal, high fiber crackers and low-fat cheese, or low-fat cottage cheese and fruit throughout the day.
Meal skipping	Establishing regular meal times is essential. Meal skipping fuels binge eating and overeating. In a time crunch, meal replacement drinks and bars can be used.
Too many liquid calories	Choose more calorie free, caffeine free, sodium free beverages (water, diet soda, unsweetened iced decaf tea)
Activities while eating	Try not to watch TV, read, or drive while eating. Distractions can cause "mindless" eating and consumption of too many calories.
Dining out often	Pre-plan ordering strategies before arrival, make healthy requests like salad dressing and sauce on the side and easy on the cheese, split entree or order $1/2$ portion sizes, or substitute steamed vegetables for french fries.

■ Developing a Diet Plan

Making small, continuous, incremental improvements in behaviors is an effective way to produce a calorie deficit and improve the overall quality of a diet. Anything the patient is willing to modify in his or her diet will be a step in the right direction. Prioritize diet issues/concerns and address them one at a time. Using a five-step behavior change plan can systematically break dietary concerns into reasonable tasks. (See Table 1.)

If a patient needs or wants a more structured diet program, you can use the exchange system to guide their food choices and portions. (See Figures 1 and 2.)

■ Providing Long-term Counseling

Food journals are self-monitoring tools used to help patients gain insight of behaviors and environmental influences contributing to weight gain. Suggest-

TABLE 1. Five Steps to Behavior Change

Step One	Identify an eating/activity behavior that is unwanted
Step Two	Identify what triggers the unwanted behavior
Step Three	Brainstorm strategies and possible solutions; generally, eliminating triggers or changing the response to them is helpful
Step Four	Try one strategy
Step Five	Evaluate the strategy: if the unwanted behavior subsides, continue practicing the strategy; if the unwanted behavior still exists, try a different strategy.

ing that patients write down what they eat everyday is a method to help them uncover food patterns. After reviewing food journals/current dietary behaviors, note the following tips for helping patients make dietary modifications.

1. Work with the patient to make sustainable, small changes in patterns and eating behaviors. Have simple and clear recommendations. It is important to aim for progress, not perfection.
2. Be positive and try to focus more on additions to diet rather than restrictions.
3. Set weight loss goals that are reasonable and achievable (10% weight loss in 6 months or 1–2 pounds per week). Discuss reward system (non-food rewards) as reinforcement for change.
4. Preplanning/meal planning is an important skill for patients to learn. Encourage pre-planning of breakfast, lunch, dinner, and snacks.
5. Patients need to know how to evaluate products in the grocery store. Label reading is a critical skill for patients to learn. Many people already try to use food labels to make decisions about food purchases, but are often times confused by the information. A comprehensive site for food label reading can be found at www.cfsan.fda.gov/~dms/food-lab.html. Shopping from a pre-planned list and not on an empty stomach helps avoid impulse purchases.
6. Cues in the environment trigger eating behavior. Keep office desks, refrigerators, and kitchen cabinets free of high-fat and high-calorie foods and instead stock up on nutritious foods. Substitute a fruit bowl for a candy dish at work, ask the waiter to remove the bread basket from the table, or take an alternative route from work to avoid passing a favorite bakery or fast-food establishment. Another cue in the environment that can stimulate eating is activities. It is best to not carry on other activities while eating like watching TV, working at a computer, or driving.
7. Healthy eating does not need to be boring and tasteless. Most of the time, patients can continue eating their favorite meals with slight recipe alterations and meal preparation changes. Suggest alterations like use low-fat versions of cheese, sour cream, and mayonnaise, cook with broth instead of oil, or use ground turkey or soy instead of ground beef.
8. Teach patients appropriate portion sizes. Tips like pre-portioning serv-

FIGURE 1.

FOOD GUIDE PYRAMID
SAMPLE FOOD CHOICE PLANS

Group	1200-1400 Calories	1400-1600 Calories	1600-1800 Calories	1800-2000 Calories	2000-2200 Calories
	Servings	Servings	Servings	Servings	Servings
Dairy	2-2	2-2	2-2	2-2	2-2
Fruit	2-3	3-3	3-5	5-5	5-5
Vegetable	3-5	5-5	5-5	5-5	5-5
Starch	6-6	6-7	7-8	8-9	9-10
Protein (Lean)	4-5	5-6	6-6	6-8	8-8
Fat	2-2	3-3	3-3	3-3	3-3

Fill in the number of servings per group to meet calorie and nutrient needs:

_____ Starch
1 serving = 80 calories
1 slice whole grain bread;
½ c. cooked pasta; 1/3 c. cooked rice
½ whole wheat bagel, english muffin
    or bun
½ c. cooked cereal; 1 oz cold cereal
1 sm. potato; ½ c. corn or peas
½ c. sweet potato

_____ Fruit
1 serving = 60 calories
1 med fruit i.e. orange, apple..
1 c. cut fruit
1/3 - ½ c. Juice
¼ c. Dried Fruit

_____ Vegetable
1 serving = 25 calories
1 c. raw leafy
½ c. raw chopped
½ c. cooked

_____ Protein
1 serving = 35-75 calories
1 oz cooked meat, poultry or fish
½ c. beans, peas, lentils
1 egg or 2 egg whites
¼ c. egg substitute
1-2 oz low fat cheese
¼ c. low fat cottage cheese

_____ Fat
1 serving = 45 calories
1 t. oil, butter, or margarine
1 T. salad dressing, sour cream
1 T. cream cheese, 2 t. peanut butter
2 T. reduced calorie salad dressing,
    sour cream or cream cheese
1 T. Seeds, 6-10 nuts, 1 sl. bacon

_____ Dairy
1 serving = 90-120 calories
1 c. low fat or nonfat milk
1 c. low fat yogurt
1 c. nonfat or low fat buttermilk

ings on a plate and not opting for seconds and not eating out of a bag or a box can help reduce quantities consumed.

9. Because more and more of the American diet is eaten at restaurants, it becomes essential that patients know how to make healthy requests from a restaurant menu. Most fast food chain restaurants have a web site disclosing nutrition information, which makes choosing healthier options possible. There are basic requests that can be made at every restaurant like "please hold the cheese," "can I have the sauce on the

FIGURE 2.

Sample 1200 Calorie Meal Plan	
Food	Food Guide Pyramid Group Servings
Breakfast:	
$\frac{1}{2}$ grapefruit	1 fruit
$\frac{1}{2}$ cup oatmeal	1 starch
$\frac{1}{2}$ bagel	1 starch
1 tsp. margarine	1 fat
1 cup skim milk	1 dairy
Lunch:	
2 oz. sliced turkey	2 protein
$\frac{1}{4}$ cup shredded cabbage	$\frac{1}{4}$ vegetable
1 tsp. Dijon mustard	free
2 slices rye bread	2 starch
1 sliced tomato/red onion	1 vegetable
with fresh squeezed lemon juice	free
$\frac{1}{2}$ cup sugar free jello	free
Snack:	
1 apple	1 fruit
Dinner:	
2 oz. broiled salmon	2 protein
1/3 cup rice	1 starch
$\frac{1}{2}$ cup steamed asparagus	1 vegetable
1 tsp. margarine	1 fat
1 mixed salad	1 vegetable
1 tablespoon fat free dressing	1 fat
$\frac{1}{2}$ cup frozen sugar free yogurt	1 dairy
Snack:	
1 slice raisin toast	1 starch
1 cup mineral water	free

side," and "can I have the vegetables instead of the fries."

10. Replace impulse snacking with planned healthy snacks like low-fat tuna salad on high fiber crackers, baked chips and low fat bean dip, or high fiber crackers with salsa and black beans. It is better to have planned snacks than have impulse snacks from a vending machine.

References

1. Putnam J and Gerrior S: Trends in the U.S. food supply, 1970-1997. USDA/ERS. Chapter 7: 133-160. http://www.ers.usda.gov/
2. Deckelbaum RJ, Fisher EA, Winston M, et al. Summary of a scientific conference on preventive nutrition: pediatrics to geriatrics. Circulation 100:450-456, 1999.
3. Executive Summary, white paper on popular weight loss diets, Jan 10, 2001. USDA. www.usda.gov

Chapter 8

Dawn Jackson, RD and Robert Kushner, MD

Commercial Programs

Commercial programs can be a useful adjunct for patients looking for additional help with their weight loss. The physician should be aware of the options available and the differences among programs. Although content and structure of commercial programs vary, they can provide education, structure, support, skills, and strategies to facilitate weight loss. Programs differ primarily by whether they offer individual counseling or group counseling, use a self-help support group model or have structured educational meetings, use a formal food plan or do not endorse any particular food plan, and whether pre-prepared food is included.

Because people's needs vary, it is important that the program directly meets their needs. No one program is right for everyone. The physician's role is to be knowledgeable about the program and work with the patient to monitor progress and provide feedback and support. Also noteworthy, the 2001 IRS ruling allows taxpayers to deduct costs for weight loss programs when prescribed by their physician to treat an existing disease.[1]

A physician can become knowledgeable about commercial programs by:

1. Asking your patient:
   - What does your weight loss plan include (portion control, prepackaged meals, weight loss drugs, liquid meals, food journals, etc.)?
   - What are your expectations from the program?
   - What are the staff credentials?
   - How does the program benefit you?
   - How often are you accountable to them?
2. Visiting the program's website or doing a peer-reviewed literature search.
3. Reviewing the Voluntary Guidelines for Providers of Weight Loss Products or Services (developed in 1998 by The Partnership for Healthy Weight Management.) The guidelines suggest that commercial programs have full disclosure on (1) program content and goals, (2) staff qualifications, (3) risks associated with the product or program, (4) program costs, and (5) outcome information on weight loss and maintenance. The guidelines are available at http://www.consumer.gov/weightloss/brochures.htm, and they provide a checklist which consumers and physicians can use to make educated decisions about commercial weight loss programs.

Below is a comparison of five popular commercial weight loss programs.

Diet: Weight Watchers® (founded in 1963)

Website address: www.weightwatchers.com

Program content: Individuals receive a budget of points to use throughout the day. Different foods are awarded different points. Individuals are budgeted an average of 18 to 35 points a day and the plan is flexible, allowing people to use their points according to individual tastes and preferences. For some people, it is easier than keeping track of calories, but it is essentially the same concept. Points are tracked in daily food journals, and regular Weight Watchers meetings are provided.

Diet composition: Dependent on how an individual budgets "points"; it is up to the individual to pick nutritious foods. Total calories range from approximately 1,200–2,200/day.

Staff qualifications: The staff is trained by the company and they are not licensed health professionals.

Risk associated with program/products: none

Cost: $15.00 registration fee; $9.95 weekly fee

Efficacy: From one to five years after weight loss period, participants regained 31.5–76.5% of weight lost. At five years: 19.4% were within 5 pounds of goal weight; 42.6% maintained a loss of 5% of their body weight or more; 18.8% maintained a loss of 10% of their body weight or more; 70.3% were below initial weight.[2]

Summary of advantages/disadvantages: It is a flexible, long-term program that can be followed easily if food journaling and point counting are done diligently.

Best for the patient who: is interested in group counseling/support, wants a structured food plan with daily record keeping, and has enough time to self-select and prepare their own meals.

Additional Reading

1. Heshka S, Greenway F, Anderson JW, et al: Self-help weight loss versus a structured commercial program after 26 weeks: a randomized controlled study. Am J Med 109:282–287, 2000.
2. Lowe MR, Miller-Kovach K, Frye N, Phelan S: An initial evaluation of commercial weight loss program: short-term effects on weight, eating behavior, and mood. Obes Res 7:51–59, 1999.
3. Weiner S: The addiction of overeating: self-help groups as treatment models. J Clin Psychol 54:163–167, 1998.

Diet: Jenny Craig®

Website address: www.jennycraig.com

Program content: There are two programs available; one program is in-center and the other via the phone. The programs offer 20-minute one-on-one consultations with a Jenny Craig counselor and exercise support with walking audiotapes. The weekly sessions emphasize an active lifestyle and healthy relationship with food. Menus are designed with pre-prepared meals that are low in calories and focus on moderation and balance. The Jenny

Craig program is based on the food-guide pyramid; menus are low in fat and cholesterol and high in fiber. The key to success on Jenny Craig comes with the transition of pre-prepared foods to self-directed, healthy meal preparation using dietary exchanges.

Diet composition: 60% carbohydrate, 20% fat, 20% protein. Total calories range from approximately 1,200–2,200/day.

Staff qualifications: Jenny Craig counselors are trained by the company and are not licensed health professionals.

Risk associated with program/products: none

Costs: Start up fees/consultation fees are between $200.00 and $370.00, pre-prepared meals average $65.00 per week, and dietary supplements are available for purchase.

Efficacy: No official data/outcome statistics have been published.

Summary of advantages/disadvantages: Pre-prepared foods make the first stages of Jenny Craig easy and convenient to follow; however, the transition stages to "real" foods and weight maintenance can be difficult.

Best for the patient who: is interested in individual weekly counseling sessions (in the center or over the phone), wants the convenience and structure of pre-prepared, calorie-controlled meals, and can afford the start-up and weekly food costs.

Additional Reading

Wolfe BL: Long-term maintenance following attainment of goal weight: a preliminary investigation. Addict Behav 17:469–477, 1992.

Diet: TOPS Club Inc.®, Take Off Weight Sensibly (founded 1948)

Website address: www.tops.org

Program content: TOPS was founded in 1948 and currently has over 9,000 chapters in the United States. The members meet weekly for weigh-ins and discuss challenges and successes. The support groups have little formal structure. The philosophy of TOPS is to use motivational competition/contests to encourage success among members. There is very little standardization between chapters. A monthly magazine ("TOPS News") tries to link all of the centers.

Diet composition: No official diet; however, diet education is based on diabetic exchange system.

Staff qualifications: Program is run by volunteers/members; no guidance from health professionals.

Risk associated with program/products: None.

Costs: $20.00 per year; book available for purchase ("the Choice is Yours") outlining American Diabetes Association's exchange system.

Efficacy: No official data/outcome statistics have been published.

Summary of advantages/disadvantages: This program is a support group with weight loss incentives; no official structured nutrition plan/diet is supported or followed by members.

Best for the patient who: is interested in group support/accountability with little dietary structure.

Additional Reading

McCall RJ, Siderits MA, Fadden TF: Differential effectiveness of informal group procedures in weight control. J Clin Psychol 33:351–360, 1977.

Diet: Overeaters Anonymous, Inc. (founded in 1960)

Website address: www.overeatersanonymous.org

Program content: Overeaters Anonymous is patterned after the 12 steps of Alcoholics Anonymous. OA is a recovery program that tries to address the emotional, spiritual, and physical aspects of overeating. OA uses literature from and based on Alcoholics Anonymous.

Diet composition: No official diet.

Staff qualifications: OA members have "sponsors"/other members to help them achieve recovery.

Risk associated with program/products: None.

Costs: No fee, although contributions are encouraged.

Efficacy: No official data/outcome statistics have been published.

Summary of advantages/disadvantages: This program is a support group with weight loss incentives; no official structured nutrition plan/diet is supported or followed by members.

Best for the patient who: is interested in group support/accountability with no dietary structure.

Additional Reading

1. Weiner S: The addiction of overeating: self-help groups as treatment models. J Clin Psychol 54:163–167, 1998.
2. Maton KI: Social support, organizational characteristics, psychological well-being, and group appraisal in three self-help group populations. Am J Community Psychol 16:53–77, 1988.
3. Yeart J: The use of Overeaters Anonymous in the treatment of eating disorders. J Psychoactive Drugs 19:303–309, 1987.

Diet: Nutrisystem.com® (founded in 1999)

Website address: www.nutrisystem.com

Program content: Nutrisystem has recently reinvented itself to become Nutrisystem.com, a primarily online weight management program. There are internet counselors for individualized sessions, personalized exercise programs, food journals, chat rooms for support, and bulletin boards online for Nutrisystem members to use (7:00 AM–2:00 AM Monday through Friday and 12:00 PM–2 AM on weekends.) Once registered, a member decides calorie level and menu plan with their Nutrisystem.com counselor. The program is designed to incorporate Nutrisystem.com's pre-prepared mail-ordered foods, but their purchase is not mandatory to be on the program.

Diet composition: 60% carbohydrates, 20% protein, 20% fat.

Staff qualifications: The on-line counselors are not health professionals, although there is a registered dietitian available to address any questions from the counselors.

Risk associated with program/products: None.

Costs: No registration fees, approximately $50.00 per week (plus shipping) for food.

Efficacy: No official data/outcome statistics have been published on Nutrisystem.com.

Summary of advantages/disadvantages: Pre-prepared foods make Nutrisystem.com easy and convenient to follow, however, the transition to "real" foods and weight maintenance can be difficult. There is no direct personal contact.

Best for the patient who: is interested in individual internet counseling sessions, wants the convenience and structure of pre-prepared, calorie-controlled meals, and does not need personal contact (program is via internet.)

Additional reading: None.

Physicians should have a working referral list of weight loss programs for their patients. Although Registered Dietitians are not considered a "commercial program," they can be an excellent resource for patients needing further counseling to achieve weight loss goals. A list of Registered Dietitians can be found at www.eatright.org

1. Http://www.obesity.org/taxguide.htm
2. Lowe MR, Miller-Kovach K, Phelan S: Weight-loss maintenance in overweight individuals one to five years following successful completion of a commercial weight loss program. Int J Obes Relat Metab Disord 25:325–331, 2001.

Chapter 9

Susan Bowerman, MS, RD

The Role of Meal Replacements in Weight Control

In a scenario all too familiar to patients and health care providers alike, a frustrated dieter complains, "I'm doing everything right . . . but I'm not losing weight!." The patient feels that he or she is counting calories and portions correctly, adhering strictly to a diet plan, but the scale does not budge. The physician, dietitian, or nutritionist gets frustrated because the reduced calorie plan *should* be working, and perhaps the patient has even brought in food records to prove that he or she is sticking with the program. What's going wrong? Inaccurate calorie counting and oversized portions are two common problems leading to weight loss failures. The use of meal replacements, which are structured to provide good nutrition within a defined calorie level, can be a valuable tool for some overweight and obese patients. While not for everyone, meal replacements can be an effective alternative to more traditional dietary approaches.

■ Problems with Portion Control and Hidden Calories

Portion control is one of the primary strategies in calorie control. But many people do not take the time to weigh and measure foods, or if they do, they abandon this practice after a period of time thinking they estimate portions fairly well. More often than not, portion sizes then gradually increase and the rate of weight loss slows. Even too much of "good" foods can impede progress, and patients are likely to underestimate their intake, even when keeping food records.

A typical diet plan specifies what foods to eat at each meal and snack, often with suggestions for substitutions in each food group to prevent boredom. Portion sizes are very specific—a cup of this, three ounces of that—and on paper, all the calories in all the portions for the day usually add up to a low calorie total. The problem comes in when people translate the diet plan into real life. Are they supposed to weigh their meat portion before or after cooking? Do they realize that a three-ounce portion of meat is the size of a deck of cards? Do they account for fats used in cooking or at the table? Do they remember that everything counts, including food eaten while standing at the sink or in the car?

How a food is prepared is also critical in keeping track of a day's intake. Many people neglect to account for fats used in cooking and at the table.

Even the most avid record-keepers often forget to account for cream in coffee, spreads on breads or vegetables, mayonnaise or cheese on sandwiches, and dressings on salads.

A few small mistakes over the course of a day or week can have a significant impact on the end result. An extra few ounces of meat could add an extra 200 calories to a day's intake. A half bagel can weigh anywhere from one ounce to three ounces, at a cost of anywhere from 75 to 225 calories. Cereals range widely in calories, from 50 calories in a cup of puffed cereal, to over 400 calories in a cup of dense granola.

Restaurant dining also poses a host of problems for dieters. Portions are almost always much larger than those specified on a meal plan, and people are often tempted to abandon diets when they eat out. The attitude is often "I paid for it, I'm going to eat it." In addition to the large portions, the method of preparation can add further calories to the meal. Hidden fats and oils, sauces, dressings, gravies, and other high fat ingredients are not always evident from the description on the menu. A restaurant Chinese chicken salad eaten in place of the 3 cups of greens, a 3-ounce chicken breast, and fat-free dressing specified in the plan could add up to a 650 calorie mistake. Table 1 illustrates how easily calories can be miscalculated.

■ Meal Replacements and Structured Foods

Meal replacements are foods that are designed to take the place of a meal while at the same time providing nutrients and good taste within a known calorie limit. These can take the form of shakes, bars, soups, or frozen portion-controlled meals, and provide the dieter with the security of knowing how many calories are being consumed at any given meal. This can be a significant advantage in avoiding costly calorie mistakes. Further, the products are usually reasonably priced and convenient to use. These special foods increase patient confidence in knowing the number of calories they are eating and reduce anxiety over making food choices. In addition, meal replacements assist patients in staying compliant with healthy behaviors.

■ Clinical Studies on Meal Replacements

Of the several hundred patients seen in our weight loss clinic, about 50% select a meal-replacement approach at the initial visit. Of those who self-select this approach, over 90% continue with the meal-replacement plan for at least 12 weeks. For weight loss, a 1,200-calorie meal plan is recommended (Table 2). This consists of meal-replacement bars or shakes substituted for two meals per day and a healthy portion-controlled dinner, which includes a salad, 2 cups steamed vegetables, and $1/2$ cup rice, pasta, or potato. Over the long term, patients can use one meal replacement per day and return to two meal replacements per day any time they begin to gain weight again.

Meal replacements have been shown to produce weight loss results superior to calorie counting. In a study by Ditschuneit et al.,[1] patients were

TABLE 1. Common Mistakes in Food Choices

If the meal plan calls for . . .	And the calories are . . .	But what is eaten is . . .	And the calories are . . .	The number of extra calories is . . .
Salad greens with 3 oz. grilled chicken and nonfat dressing	360	Restaurant Chinese Chicken Salad	1014	654
1 cup whole grain pasta with 1 cup tomato sauce	260	2 cups pasta with 1 cup alfredo sauce	600	340
1 cup flaked cereal with 1 cup nonfat milk	170	1 cup granola with 1 cup 2% milk	570	400
Sandwich with two slices whole grain bread, three ounces of turkey, mustard, lettuce, and tomato	295	Sandwich with two slices white bread, five ounces of roast beef, mayonnaise, lettuce and tomato	520	225
3 small pancakes	240	4 large pancakes	610	370
1 medium baked potato with fresh chives and 1 tablespoon fat-free ranch dressing	250	1 large "stuffed" baked potato	740	490
TOTAL	1575	TOTAL	4054	2479

TABLE 2. 1200-Calorie Meal Plan

Breakfast:	Meal Replacement + a piece of Fruit
Lunch:	Meal Replacement + large green salad with fat-free dressing + a piece of Fruit
Afternoon Snack:	Piece of fruit or raw vegetables or meal replacement snack bar
Dinner:	Prepared Frozen Dinner Large green salad with fat-free dressing 2 cups of steamed vegetables $1/_2$ cup brown rice or whole grain pasta, or 1 small baked potato with skin Fruit for dessert

divided into two groups. One group counted calories, consuming between 1200 and 1500 calories per day. The second group used two meal replacements as part of an overall diet plan of 1200 to 1500 calories. The calorie-counting group lost approximately three pounds over the first 12 weeks, while the meal replacement group lost approximately 17 pounds. The markedly increased weight loss in the meal replacement group can be attributed to the enhanced dietary compliance mediated by the use of meal replacements. Both groups were then given one meal replacement per day over two years and both groups lost additional weight. Ditschuneit and colleagues have shown that this approach can be maintained for up to four years.[2]

In a 1994 study, 300 men and women at six sites throughout the United States took two meal replacement shakes/day as part of a 1200 cal/day diet plan for 12 weeks. For the next 24 months, they consumed one shake per day as part of a 1200-calorie diet plan. Weight loss was about 7% of the starting weight, and those subjects who continued to the end of the study (approximately 56% of the initial group) maintained much of their weight loss.[3]

Recent research has demonstrated that with the exception of fruits and vegetables, increased variety of intake in all categories of foods promotes obesity.[4] By reducing variety, meal replacements help patients maintain a structured diet and portion control. Many of these meal replacements are excellent sources of protein, fiber, vitamins, and minerals (including calcium), and may be superior to simply restricting conventional food intake, which could cause nutritional adequacy.

■ Meal Plans Using Meal Replacements

Most meal replacements and frozen portion-controlled meals contain 300 calories or fewer. By rounding out the meal with vegetables, salads, and fruit for dessert, a nutritious and satisfying meal contains roughly 450 calories. Table 2 shows a sample 1200-calorie menu which utilizes meal replacements twice a day. The meals are supplemented with a fruit at breakfast and with vegetables and salad at lunch and dinner, with a fruit for dessert. Since many people complain that preparing the proper foods for a weight loss diet is too time consuming, the simplicity of this plan appeals to many because the meal replacement takes care of the entrée. Adding the vegetables and fruits can be simplified, too. Whole pieces of fruit, precut melons, prewashed salad greens and carrots, and washed and cut vegetables ready for steaming are all widely available in most supermarkets. A variety of fat-free salad dressings and seasoned vinegars complete the shopping list. If the average person eats 21 meals and 14 snacks per week, replacing ten meals per week with a structured meal replacement can result in significant calorie control.

■ Why Suggest Meal Replacements?

Meal replacements can be an easy-to-use teaching tool for the busy health care provider. Diet plans incorporating meal replacements are easy to review with patients and easy for patients to grasp. Their convenience, availability, and pricing make a good choice for today's busy lifestyles. The entire day's meal plan should incorporate whole fresh fruits and vegetables and whole grains to provide phytonutrients, vitamins, minerals and fiber. Using a daily multiple vitamin/mineral supplement is also appropriate.

In counseling patients on the use of meal replacements, the health care provider can stress their value to the patient. For many patients, the simplicity of the meal plan takes the guesswork out of counting calories and macronutrients. It is important to stress to the patient that meal replacements can provide good nutrition and can provide a healthy alternative to skipping meals.

■ What to Look for in a Meal Replacement

In counseling patients, advise them to select a meal replacement shake, bar, soup, or frozen meal with 300 calories or fewer. That way, fruits and vegetables can be added to the meal and the calories will still be within reason. Fat calories ideally should be no more than 20% of total calories. Most shakes, bars, and soups will be much lower than this, but advise patients to read labels carefully on frozen meals. The shakes, bars, and soups should provide vitamins, minerals, and fiber. Most importantly, suggest that patients taste several meal replacements until they find the ones they prefer.

■ Summary

In counseling overweight and obese patients, the primary care provider can easily explain the value of the use of meal replacements in maintaining control over their calorie intake. The diet plan is simple, yet effective, and patients will be encouraged by the results they achieve. You will find that many of your patients are helped by this approach, and that you will be rewarded in the process with better patient satisfaction and retention.

References

1.   Ditschuneit HH, Flechtner-Mors M, Johnson, TD et al: Metabolic and weight loss effects of a long-term dietary intervention in obese patients. Am J Clin Nutr 69:198–204, 1999.
2.   Ditschuneit HH, Frier H, Fletchner-Mors M, Greene H: Metabolic and weight loss effects of long-term dietary intervention in obese patients: four-year results. Obes Res 8(5):399–402, 2000.
3.   Heber D, Ashley JM, Wang HJ, et al: Clinical evaluation of a minimal intervention meal replacement regimen for weight reduction. J Am Coll Nutr 13:608–614, 1994.
4.   Roberts S: Multiple Components Contribute to Dietary Risk for Obesity (abstract). Obesity Res 7(Suppl 1):13S, 1999.

Chapter 10

Daniel H. Bessesen, MD

Talking to Patients About Popular Diet Books

With the recent increase in the prevalence of obesity, there has been an associated dramatic rise in the number of diet books published. A recent search of books on Amazon.com using the key words 'weight loss' returned 1214 matches. Of the top 50 best-selling diet books, almost 60% were published in 1999 or 2000.[1] Most clinicians have had the experience of a patient coming to the office asking for advice about one of these diets. What should the clinician do when encountering one of these patients? Should he or she advocate the diet? Dissuade the individual from attempting these diets? Recommend any of these books to patients?

These books frequently have a similar style and structure. The structure has three general parts. The first part is a description of the advocate of the diet. The advocate is generally the author, although many of these authors have had help from professional writers. For many or most of these books the author relates a compelling personal story to the reader. The reader gets the feeling that the author is speaking directly to him or her. The author is portrayed as having had an experience of enlightenment or discovery that gave them insight into the basic cause of obesity or central problem with the typical diet. The author may be portrayed as a renegade or rebel, bucking commonly held notions about diet and health. The author says he knows something that others do not know. The reader believes that the author truly wants to help with this newly found knowledge.

The second part of the book is this central idea or concept. The concept is pitched to the reader as being new. Usually the concept sounds scientific and it is linked to some form of research. Usually it is a concept that is distinct from and even contrary to the usual advice given to patients by doctors and professional organizations such as the American Heart Association, American Diabetes Association, or U.S. Department of Agriculture (USDA). The concept is usually simple, can be stated in one or two sentences, and understood by virtually anyone. The author usually argues that, "if only this important idea were more broadly accepted then people's health and weight would improve." At this point, if the reader is engaged, he or she believes that the author has his or her best interests at heart, and that the author has some new understanding that others do not yet have that will now be shared with the reader. This is the foundation on which the reader may then embark on behavior change.

The third part of the program is the diet itself. The diet is an outgrowth of the central concept of the book. These diets can be grouped into several broad categories based on their nutritional approach. The Atkin's Diet[5] is a high-fat, low carbohydrate diet. The Zone Diet[8] is a moderate-fat, high-protein diet. Other moderate fat diets include *Sugar Buster's*[6] and some of the diets in the *Eat Right for Your Type*[7] book. Several recent books written by respected researchers in the field of nutrition take a more balanced approach with regards to macronutrient composition. An the other end of the spectrum are the very-low-fat diets advocated by Dr. Dean Ornish[4] and Dr. Pritikin.[3] Following is a review of the details of several of these popular diet books.

The Atkins Diet[5]

The Advocate. Dr. Atkins was trained as a physician and cardiologist. The strength of his advocacy comes from his assertion that he has personally cared for thousands of overweight individuals and that his direct, personal clinical experience treating patients forms the basis of his diet program. He does not argue that he is a scientific expert or nutritional researcher. He argues that the success of the diet has been proven to him through his work with patients.

The Concept. The central concept in the Atkins Diet is that carbohydrate stimulates insulin secretion, which in turn stimulates appetite. Dr. Atkins argues that a low fat/high carbohydrate diet is doomed to failure because people are constantly hungry because of high insulin levels. He believes that by severely restricting carbohydrate in the diet producing a state of "benign dietary ketosis," the individual can continue to eat good-tasting foods, experience little or no hunger, and lose weight more rapidly then they would on a lower fat diet. In fact, he seems to argue that people will lose weight on a high fat diet without really restricting calories. His focus is very much on restricting carbohydrate without any reference really to accounting total caloric intake. He seems to believe that it is a myth that caloric restriction is necessary for weight loss.

The Diet. As practiced this is a very-low-carbohydrate, high-fat diet. It has an induction phase during which time total daily intake of carbohydrates is limited to 20 g. During the maintenance phase this is liberalized to 40 g. Other than this careful restriction of carbohydrate, there are few restrictions in the diet. Likewise, there is no need to count calories, making the diet fairly easy to follow. The result of these recommendations is a diet high in fat, often high in saturated fat, and low in calories. In fact the induction diet is roughly a 1200 kcal/day diet.

The Data. Perhaps the strongest data in support of this diet are the estimated twenty million plus people world wide who have either read Dr. Atkins book or contacted his website. In truth there has been very little research on either the effectiveness or risks of this diet. The details of research which has been done on this diet were outlined in a recent issue of Obesity Research.[1] These studies showed that the high-fat diet advocated by Dr. Atkins does appear to cause dietary ketosis. In addition, it does appear to cause relatively rapid short-term weight loss that is the result of both moderate caloric restriction and loss of water weight due to the consumption of glycogen stores. There is modest evidence that this diet is associated with mild reductions in blood lipids, although the data is too limited to form firm conclusions. The improvements in blood lipids seen are likely due to the hypocaloric nature of the diet and the accompanying weight loss. Virtually any state of weight loss is associated with improvement in lipid levels. Some have been concerned that this diet is nutritionally inadequate. A careful analysis of the foods and quantities consumed during induction and maintenance diet does indeed suggest that the Atkins Diet is deficient in a number of vitamins and minerals. However, the evidence in support of this point is not large.

Some have been concerned that the severe carbohydrate restriction in the Atkins program may result in a decline in exercise tolerance. However, studies examining this issue suggest that individuals actually seem to adapt to prolonged ketosis and that a high-fat diet does not seem to adversely affect maximal or submaximal exercise performance in untrained individuals.

While anecdotal evidence does suggest that the Atkins Diet may be associated with a rapid initial weight loss largely due to mobilization of glycogen stores and an increased sense of satiety during the weight loss phase, long-term data on the effects of this diet are not available. It may be that for some individuals this diet program does provide a more effective way of losing weight. However there are many questions about the long-term health effects of high intakes of saturated fat. Additionally, there are concerns that people may not be able to sustain this diet over a period of many years. Recent review of the National Weight Control Registry (see chapter 17) suggests that very few people who have succeeded in maintaining weight loss long term are using the Atkins program.

The Zone Diet[8]

The Advocate. Dr. Barry Sears holds a Ph.D. degree. He describes his research in the area of eicosanoid biology, and details the importance of eicosanoids in maintaining health. He describes his work providing nutritional guidance to high performance athletes on a number of competitive intercollegiate teams. While not a recognized nutrition researcher or an experienced clinician, he comes from a scientific background.

The Concept. Dr. Sears argues that the our bodies developed systems for assimilating nutrients during the hunter-gatherer stage of human evolution. He suggests that the current recommendations for high-carbohydrate, low-fat diets are not reflective of the kind of diets eaten by hunter-gatherers. He believes that to optimize health we should consume an ideal ratio of protein, carbohydrate, and fat, and that 30% protein, 30% fat, and 40% carbohydrate is the optimal ratio. He suggests that nutrients are like drugs and that they have dose-response curves. Too much dietary carbohydrate would produce too high a concentration of insulin. Too little carbohydrate would produce excessive counter-regulatory hormones and too little insulin.

The Diet. Dr. Sears puts a strong emphasize on protein intake. This is really the starting point for his diet. He encourages increased intakes of protein-rich, low-fat food sources including chicken, fish, and tofu. He encourages a moderate intake of fruits and vegetables. The third component of the diet is to modestly restrict carbohydrate. This is a moderate-fat, high-protein diet.

The Data. Dr. Sears has included in his book anecdotal data about the effectiveness of his diet from his work with elite athletes. He also provides evidence in support of his ideas about eicosanoid biology. However, he does not provide evidence that his diet helps overweight adults lose weight. In fact this diet is not specifically designed as a weight-loss diet. It is primarily designed as a diet to "optimize health." While he does argue that some people will lose weight on this diet, that is not the primary goal of the diet and obese individuals are not the primary target of this book.

While the concept that nutrients have dose-response curves is an attractive idea, and the idea that our diet differs from the hunter-gatherer diet is probably true, there is little information available to support the use of this diet. There is modest evidence in those with preexisting renal failure and those with diabetes complicated by renal disease that high protein intakes may adversely effect renal function. However, for an individual with normal renal function there does not currently exist conclusive evidence that high-protein intakes are harmful. There is moderate evidence that protein may be more satiating calorie for calorie then either carbohydrate or fat, and this evidence supports the notion that high protein diets may be useful in promoting weight loss. There are concerns that the sole emphasis in this diet is placed on the ratio of macronutrients. There are commercial products available that conform to the 30/30/40 ratio which contain only 30% fat, however most of that is saturated fat. High intake of saturated fat is associated with increases in LDL cholesterol and is probably associated with increased risk of heart disease.

Eat Right for Your Type[7]

The Advocate. Dr. Peter D'Adamo is a naturopathic physician whose father was also a naturopathic physician. The younger Dr. D'Adamo emphasizes that he is bringing the discovery made by his father many years ago to the reader today, the idea that different people should eat different diets. He conveys his personal experiences watching his father help individuals improve their health by optimizing their diet for their personal biology. Dr. D'Adamo does not appear to have any formal advanced training in the biologic sciences or traditional western medicine. He received his naturopathic studies degree from John Bastyr College in Seattle.

The Concept. The fundamental idea espoused by Dr. D'Adamo is that when expert organizations advise one diet for all people they lose sight of the fact that different people probably respond differently to different diets. He argues that blood type will provide useful information on how an individual will respond to a particular diet. He suggests that there is a different optimal diet for people of different blood types, and that the basis for these differences comes from genetic backgrounds of people with different blood types. He believes that people with specific blood types represent different "stages in human evolution." In addition, he believes that the blood type determines immune responses to particular components of the diet.

The Diet. The book is divided into different sections for different blood types. For example, type A blood is called the "the cultivator." He argues that type A individuals flourish on vegetarian diets because of their genetic background. Blood type O diet he calls "the hunter" diet. These individuals he believes require a high protein/high meat intake while restricting consumption of grains, breads, and other carbohydrates. He goes into detail about the specific diet plan for each blood type, as well as associated personality traits and adverse health effects and health benefits of dietary change in each blood type.

The Data. The idea that different people respond differently to the same dietary intervention is an idea that is receiving increased scientific attention. High carbohydrate diets have been shown to produce high triglyceride levels in a subset of individuals. High intakes of simple sugar may promote insulin resistance in "carbohydrate sensitive" individuals. It may be very important to consider how an individual's genotype interacts with particular components in the diet to produce good or bad health effects.

However, the evidence used to link blood type with these predispositions is not strong. Modern nutrition researchers have not embraced the idea that blood type can define susceptibility to particular diet types. Likewise, the scientific evidence supporting the link between food lectins and immune responses is weak. Finally, Dr. D'Adamo does not present any prospective randomized scientifically reviewed interventional studies that support his ideas, nor have other investigators used these diets in a systematic manner to evaluate the validity of the claims made in the book.

Volumetrics[9]

The Advocate. Dr. Barbara Rolls is a respected researcher in the area of satiety and food intake in humans. She has conducted carefully controlled studies on satiety using careful weigh and measure methods to quantitate food intake in human subjects. She has published these results in peer-reviewed scientific journals, and she has broad credibility in the scientific community. However, she is not a full-time clinician experienced in treating obese patients. Her views largely come from her research background.

The Concept. While the focus in many mainstream diets has been on restricting dietary fat, Dr. Rolls studies have shown her that it is not the fat content that promotes overeating but rather the energy density of foods. She has conducted studies where the fat content, carbohydrate content, or energy density were varied independently and food intake measured. She found that human subjects tend to overeat on diets that contain high energy density (cal/gram of food). While in general high fat foods have a high energy density, some high carbohydrate foods also have high energy density. Conversely, there are relatively high fat foods which can be made to have a low energy density. The things that lower energy density in foods include water and fiber. The concept of the book is that individuals will feel full and reduce calories if they can consume foods that have a low energy density.

The Diet. The diet contains foods that are high in fiber or high in water, including fruits, vegetables, and liquid foods.

The Data. The studies performed by Dr. Rolls clearly show that over the short term (hours to days) human subjects tend to overeat foods with high energy density. However, currently there is little evidence from interventional studies demonstrating the effectiveness of low-energy-density diets. While it seems reasonable that these diets would have beneficial effects, this idea simply has not been broadly tested and validated in relevant populations. The specific people who will respond to the diet, the health effects, and the ability of this diet to produce long-term maintenance of a reduced weight are not known at this time.

The Glucose Revolution[10]

The Advocates. This is a recent book by Jennie Brand-Miller and Thomas Wolever, two nutrition researchers who have been interested in the glycemic index for many years. Both have done studies examining the health effects of diets that vary in glycemic index. In this book the authors hope to popularize the idea of the glycemic index and provide readers with information on which they can construct their own diets with a low glycemic index. While the scientific foundation of these authors is good, they do not come from a background of treating overweight or obese patients. Their ideas grow out of experimental studies in humans.

The Concept. The central idea of this book is that a low glycemic index diet will promote weight loss, improve athletic performance, manage diabetes, and reduce the risk of heart disease. The glycemic index is a concept based on the observation that different forms of carbohydrate produce varying glucose and insulin responses following ingestion. In the past it was thought that the complex carbohydrates were more slowly absorbed than simple sugars. However, experimental studies conducted by Dr. Wolever and others have shown that in fact many starch-containing foods such as potatoes and white bread have a greater glycemic excursion than equal amounts of simple sugars. These investigators have characterized a large number of foods and found that there is a broad range of glycemic and insulin excursions following ingestion, which they have cataloged. These relationships are complex, however. The glycemic index of a particular food is influenced by the other foods that are eaten with it, as well as other factors such as method of preparation. Currently, it is difficult to obtain reliable information about the glycemic index of commonly eaten foods. This lack of information has made it difficult for consumers to actually use this concept in constructing their own diets. This book then provides information and background on which a consumer can construct a low glycemic index diet.

The Diet. The diet advocated by these authors is a low glycemic index diet. They suggest a variety of food substitutions, which would convert a typical American diet to a lower glycemic index diet.

The Data. There is no question that different forms of carbohydrate produce different levels of glucose excursion following ingestion. In addition, there is increasing evidence that a low glycemic index diet might have beneficial health effects. However, there are no long-term prospective interventional studies that show that this kind of diet will produce sustained weight loss. There are epidemiologic studies that support some of the claims made by these authors. However, there are problems with focusing only on the glycemic index as a marker of a healthy diet. For example, some foods that have a low glycemic index might be high in simple sugars because sucrose and fructose have a low glycemic index. An oat bran muffin has a glycemic index of 60, while frosted flakes has a glycemic index of 55. Consumers then might think that choosing Frosted Flakes would be a more healthy food choice than an oat bran muffin. Other foods that are high in fat, even high in saturated fat, have a very low glycemic index. M&M's chocolate peanuts have a glycemic index of 33. The result is that a consumer could selectively comb through the list of foods, and find foods that they enjoyed eating that had low glycemic index which more traditional nutritional recommendations would suggest are not good for their health.

The Ornish Diet[4]

The Advocate. Dr. Dean Ornish received his M.D. from Baylor. He has trained at some of the best medical institutions in the country, and has approached his nutritional research with the goal of testing his diet and lifestyle program with the same rigorous standards that would be applied to any new medical therapy. He began his program with the belief that heart disease was primarily a lifestyle disease. He believed that rather than treating atherosclerosis with medications and surgery, lifestyle modifications, including a low-fat vegetarian diet, meditation, and exercise, could be an effective alternative. Perhaps more than some other diet programs, Dr. Ornish's program is an outgrowth both of careful research and clinical experience. However, his clinical experience takes place in a very specialized environment where wealthy patients have come to seek highly individualized attention. Many think that this type of program is not well suited for the constraints present in the typical primary care practice.

The Concept. The Ornish program is not primarily a weight loss program. Neither is it primarily a diet that stands alone. Rather this program was conceived as a treatment for coronary artery disease. Treatment involves dietary modification along with yoga-based exercise, meditation, and group support. The success of the program in preventing coronary artery disease prompted Dr. Ornish to propose the diet as a weight-loss program, perhaps motivated in part by the pervasiveness of the problem.

The Diet. The diet is an extremely low fat (10%) vegetarian diet which is an outgrowth of the older Pritikin Diet.[3] While the Pritikin Diet allowed some meat consumption, the Ornish diet does not. This diet minimizes virtually all fats in cooking and food preparation.

The Data. This program has been extensively studied, and the results published in outstanding medical journals. The studies demonstrate that this program is an effective way to produce modest improvements in coronary artery disease in those with established atherosclerosis. These studies have also demonstrated modest sustained weight loss in the same subjects. The lipid profiles in these individuals have shown moderate reductions in LDL cholesterol; however, there are modest rises in serum triglyceride levels. The subjects in these studies have been highly motivated patients with known coronary artery disease. This diet program has not been tested in a large group of overweight individuals, neither is Dr. Ornish primarily experienced in caring for overweight or obese patients. Some have been concerned that extremely high carbohydrate diets might promote increased triglyceride levels in some susceptible individuals. Most feel that the extreme fat restriction and vegetarian nature of the diet make this program unattractive and even unrealistic for most Americans.

Sugar Busters[6]

The Advocates. This book is authored by four individuals, three of whom are physicians and one of whom is a CEO of a Fortune 500 Energy Company. The principal author, Mr. H. Leighton Steward, really aims to share his personal experience practicing a diet which he adapted from an older book entitled Sugars Blues, by William Dufty. It seems that this author believed a diet low in refined carbohydrates was helpful to him, but that previous diet books were overly technical. His goal seems to be to share the benefits of this sugar-restricted diet with others using language that is not overly technical. None of the authors has been formally trained in nutrition, is actively involved in nutritional research, or appears to be actively involved in the clinical care of overweight or obese patients.

The Concept. The central idea of this book is that the typical American diet is harmful because it contains high amounts of simple sugars and refined carbohydrates. The effects of this diet are that these simple sugars raise glucose and insulin levels, producing an accumulation of fat tissue. The authors argue that the sugar is turned into fat. They argue that removing sugar and refined carbohydrate from the diet will prevent heart disease, improve glucose levels, and promote sustained weight loss.

The Diet. The authors refer to the glycemic index; however, this is not discussed in any depth, and is not the basis of the diet. The diet promotes increased consumption of fruits, vegetables, and whole-grain foods. It discourages the consumption of simple sugars and refined carbohydrates.

The Data. There is no data that this particular diet plan has any advantages over the diets advocated by the USDA, the American Heart Association, or other organizations. These authors do not seem interested in doing any research to demonstrate the effectiveness of this diet. In fact, many of the statements that they make are not supported by the available scientific literature. Specifically, the glycemic indexes of sucrose and fructose (both simple sugars) have been measured and are in fact lower than those of most other carbohydrates. Therefore the central contention that simple sugars are harmful because they cause wide swings in blood sugar is simply not supported by studies in this area. Second, the authors contention that carbohydrate is "turned into fat" is also not supported by scientific studies. The process of de novo lipogenesis has been extensively studied and appears to be a minor biochemical pathway. It is possible that consumption of high carbohydrate diets promotes the storage of dietary fat; however, the idea that a substantial portion of dietary carbohydrate is actually converted into triglyceride simply is not supported by careful research. It seems that the attraction of this book stands largely from its simple language, positive tone, and large type.

■ What Approach Should Be Taken?

Most primary care providers are faced frequently with patients who are interested in pursuing one of these diet programs. There are three general approaches that could be taken: discourage patients from using any of these diets: advocate and promote one of these diet plans, or support the patient in whatever their goals are, while discussing potential problems with each of these diet plans.

Discouraging patients from participating in these programs is perhaps the easiest thing to do, and is likely the most common response. With the exception of the Ornish Diet, none of these diets has been tested in randomized controlled interventional trials and shown to be effective. None are supported by reputable organizations such as the USDA, the American Heart Association, the American Diabetes Association, or other groups interested in healthy eating. Some of the ideas which underlie these diets are simply wrong as outlined above. Some of these diets may be actually harmful. It is possible that the high saturated fat intake of the Atkins Diet may promote atherosclerosis. There is evidence that the Atkins diet is deficient in a number of vitamins and micronutrients. There is some concern that the Ornish diet may cause some nutritional deficiencies. However, when a patient comes to the office ready to try one of these diets, he or she has already progressed through precontemplative and contemplative stages and is ready for action (see chapter 6). It seems unfortunate to undermine an individual who is motivated and attempting to take responsibility for their health. There are elements of truth within many of these diets. It is true that many patients have trouble adhering to a high carbohydrate/low fat diet. It is probably true that individuals who are ketotic experience less hunger. It is true that there is objective evidence that a low glycemic index diet is beneficial to health. The Ornish Diet has been extensively studied and health benefits have been shown for those with coronary artery disease. The research of Dr. Rolls has clearly shown that energy density is related to satiety. And so it seems unreasonable to discount these diets out of hand.

An alternative approach would be to pick one of these diets and support it. But which to choose? None of these diets has been proven better than the others. Sometimes a care provider will have a positive experience with a particular diet and then simply advocate this diet for others. The arguments for any one of these diets are made in the book, and the practitioner can simply reinforce and reiterate these arguments. The diets are clearly outlined in the books as are shopping lists and sample menus and recipes. However, given the lack of data and lack of acceptance for these diets in the general medical community, this does not seem to be advisable.

The option that many practitioners use then is to learn about these diets, and support their patients in the choices they are making. Many patients are excited about the diet when they start, but the physician needs to help them look forward to the period of weight maintenance, and the possibility of relapse, providing objective information about the health effects of the diet, including measures of weight loss, BMI, waist circumference, lipid, glucose and insulin levels, and adequacy of vitamin intakes. If an individual on one of these diets is losing weight and seeing improvements in blood pressure, insulin, glucose, and lipids, then it may reasonable to continue supporting the patient with that diet. If the individual is not experiencing health benefits then the physician can work with him or her to decide what alternative strategy might be more successful.

One problem with all of these books is that they are written from a point of view that "experts are wrong." Each book promotes its author as the sole purveyor of accurate nutritional information. However, as more books are written with more and more individuals challenging the traditional dogma of a low-fat, high-carbohydrate diet high in vegetables and fruits, the general public is reaching a state of confusion about who to believe and what to eat. In addition, many patients experience resistance when talking to their primary care providers about these diets. The result is that they are left alone to make decisions about the accuracy of the information that they are receiving. It might be better for the patient to have an advocate in his or her own health care provider. There is something to learn from many of these books. Perhaps some patients need a motivator and an advocate. Perhaps we can learn that individuals need a simple clear message to motivate them. In addition, perhaps people want to feel that their health care provider has their best interest at heart. By supporting patients in the long-term management of overweight and obesity, learning from these many authors while not overestimating the benefits of these diets, hopefully patients and healthcare providers can reach some individualized long-term nutritional strategies that will benefit health.

References

1. Freedman MR, King J, Kennedy E: Popular Diets: Scientific Review. Obesity Research 9(S1):1S-40S2
2. Ornish D: Eat More, Weigh Less. New York, Harper Paper Backs, 1993.

3. Pritikin R: The Pritikin Principle. Alexandria, VA, Time Life Books, 2000
4. Ornish D: Dr. Dean Ornish's Program for Reversing Heart Disease. New York, Ballantine Books, 1990.
5. Atkins RC: Dr. Atkins New Diet Revolution. New York, Avon Books, Incorporated., 1992.
6. Steward HP, Bethea NC, Andrews SS Balart LA: Sugar Busters! New York, Ballantine Books, 1995.
7. D'Adamo PJ,Whitney C: Eat Right for Your Type. New York, GP Putnam's Sons, 1996.
8. Sears B, Lawren B: Enter the Zone. New York, Harper Collins, 1995.
9. Rolls B, Barnett RA: The Volumetrics Weight-Control Plan. New York, Harper Collins, 2000.
10. Brand-Miller J, Wolever TMS, Colagiuri S, Foster-Powell K: The Glucose Revolution. New York, Marlowe & Company, 1996.

Chapter 11

Robert Kushner, MD

Very-Low-Calorie Diets

Very-low-calorie diets (VLCDs) can be a useful option for patients needing rapid weight loss for medical or behavioral/lifestyle reasons. In general, VLCDs are characterized by the following four features: (1) are 800 kcal or less per day; (2) are relatively enriched in protein (0.8 to 1.5 gm/kg of ideal body weight per day); (3) are designed to include the full complement of the dietary reference intake (RDI) for vitamins, minerals, electrolytes, and fatty acids; and (4) are intended to completely replace usual food intake. Due to their substantial caloric restriction and associated risks, VLCDs are typically prescribed for only 12 to 16 weeks under direct medical supervision. Patients can expect an average loss of 1.5 to 2.0 kg/week in women and 2.0 to 2.5 kg/week in men, with average total losses of 20 kg over 12 weeks. Although VLCDs produce greater initial weight loss than low calorie diets (800-1500 kcal), long-term results are not substantially different. In a study by Wadden and Frey, one half of patients maintained losses of 5% or more and one third losses of 10% or more at 3 years following a 12-week VLCD treatment.[1]

VLCD products are formulated by the manufacturer as ready-to-drink supplements, powders (which are reconstituted with water to make a beverage shake), or foods and bars (Table 1). Patients typically drink 5 supplements each day along with 64 ounces of non-caloric fluids. Some 'modified' programs include adding small amounts of lean meat and low calorie vegetables as well. The products are distributed through and supervised by physicians who have experience in managing patients on VLCDs. For physicians interested in incorporating VLCDs into their weight management practice, some of the manufacturers offer a range of support options, including the product, patient and physician materials, an operations manual, and a central database for tracking outcomes. VLCDs should provide instructions on behavior modification and exercise to enhance initial and long-term results, either in small groups or individually.

According to a review by the National Task Force on the Prevention and Treatment of Obesity,[2] indications for initiating a VLCD include well-motivated individuals who are moderately to severely obese (BMI > 30), have failed at more conservative approaches to weight loss, and have a medical condition that would be immediately improved with rapid weight loss. These conditions include uncontrolled type 2 diabetes, hypertriglyceridemia, obstructive sleep apnea, and symptomatic peripheral edema. Contraindications to VLCD's include systemic infections or diseases causing

TABLE 1. Very-Low-Calorie Diets

Product	Manufacturer
HMR shakes: 500, 70+, 800, soups HMR entrees HMR bars	Health Management Resources, Boston, MA 617-357-9876 www.yourbetterhealth.com
Optifast 800 shakes: ready-to-make powder Soups Bars	Novartis, Minneapolis, MN 1-800-662-2540 www.optifast.com
Medifast shakes: 55, 70, +	Healthrite, Owings Mills, MD 1-800-638-7867 www.medifast.net

protein wasting, unstable cardiac or cerebrovascular disease, acute and chronic renal failure, severe or end-stage liver disease, and psychiatric disorders that may interfere with patient adherence.

All patients need to undergo a comprehensive history and physical examination along with laboratory testing for a complete blood count, general chemistry profile, urinalysis, and ECG before undertaking a VLCD. Most often patients sign an informed consent form clearly outlining the risks and benefits of the treatment. Adverse reactions may include fatigue or weakness, dizziness, constipation, hair loss, dry skin, nausea, diarrhea, change in menses, and cold intolerance. More serious complications include development of gout, gallstones, and cardiac disturbances. The physician and support staff needs to continuously monitor patients for these side effects and adjust treatment accordingly. For patients with a history of gout or hyperuricemia, prophylactic treatment with an antigout agent (allopurinol, probenecid, or colchicine) should be considered. The risk for gallstone formation increases exponentially at rates of weight loss above 1.5 kg/week.[3] Prophylaxis against gallstone formation with ursodeoxycholic acid, 600 mg/day, is effective in reducing this risk.[4] Periodic ECG monitoring for prolongation of the QT interval or development of dysrhythmias should also be performed as long as the patient remains on the VLCD.

References

1. Wadden TA, Frey DL:A multicenter evaluation of a proprietary weight loss program or the treatment of marked obesity: a five-year follow-up. Int J Eat Disord 22:203–212, 1997.
2. National Task Force on the Prevention and Treatment of Obesity: Very low-calorie diets. JAMA 270:967–974, 1993.
3. Weinsier RL, Wilson LJ, Lee J: Medically safe rate of weight loss for the treatment of obesity: a guideline based on risk of gallstone formation. Am J Med 98:115–117, 1995.
4. Shiffman ML, Kaplan GD, Brinkman-Kaplan V, Vickers FF: Prophylaxis against gallstone formation with ursodeoxycholic acid in patients participating in a very-low-calorie diet program. Ann Intern Med 122:899–905, 1995.

Chapter 12

John M. Jakicic, PhD, and Kara I. Gallagher, PhD

Physical Activity Considerations for Management of Body Weight

The management of body weight can be very complex. However, in the simplest terms, the balance between energy intake and energy expenditure determines weight gain, weight maintenance, or weight loss. There are three general components of energy expenditure: resting energy expenditure, the thermic effect of a meal, and energy expenditure in the form of physical activity. Of these three components, energy expenditure from physical activity is the most variable and provides the greatest opportunity for interventions to modify total energy expenditure. The following is a summary of the role of physical activity in the management of body weight, recommendations for physical activity in managing body weight, and strategies for enhancing participation in physical activity in patients within a primary care setting.

■ The Benefits of Physical Activity

Physical activity in the form of regular exercise appears to be a key factor in the management of body weight and the treatment of chronic conditions typically associated with obesity. While it is clear that changes in dietary intake may have the greatest impact on body weight over the short-term, the addition of physical activity to a dietary program has been shown to enhance weight loss. Moreover, adequate physical activity has been shown to be one of the best predictors of long-term maintenance of weight loss and the prevention of weight gain in adults. Therefore, weight management interventions should include an appropriate physical activity program, and guidelines for developing this type of program are discussed below.

In addition to playing a significant role in the management of body weight, exercise offers benefits that are independent of changes in body weight. It has been shown that increases in physical activity typically result in improvements in cardiorespiratory fitness. Results of longitudinal studies have shown that increased levels of cardiorespiratory fitness reduce the relative risk for all-cause morbidity and mortality independent of body weight and other potential confounding factors.[3,12,16] This is significant because these findings appear to indicate that overweight adults can improve their health through increasing fitness regardless of whether they can successfully reduce their body weight.

Physical activity may be effective for reducing morbidity and mortality because of its impact on a number of risk factors that appear to be common in overweight and obese adults. It has been suggested that obesity can increase the likelihood of developing hypertension, hypertriglyceridemia, hyperglycemia, and hyperinsulinemia. Numerous studies have been conducted which demonstrate that physical activity can be an effective treatment for these conditions. Exercise can reduce resting blood pressure, triglycerides, and blood glucose, while increasing high-density lipoprotein cholesterol and insulin sensitivity. Thus, overweight adults should be encouraged to engage in adequate levels of physical activity to control body weight and reduce potential risk factors that may be present.

In summary, low levels of fitness and numerous health-related risk factors are common in overweight and obese adults. There is evidence that interventions targeted at increasing physical activity can have a significant impact on long-term weight management. In addition, increasing physical activity can improve cardiorespiratory fitness, which has been linked to reductions in morbidity and mortality rates. Therefore, interventions conducted within the primary care setting to increase physical activity can have a significant impact on the health of overweight and obese adults.

■ Methods of Assessing Activity Patterns

Prior to developing a physical activity program for patients, it is important to understand their current physical activity patterns. Within the 10- to 15-minute office visit there is not sufficient time to conduct a lengthy interview focusing on this one health behavior. Thus, a physical activity history can be completed by the patient prior to being seen by the physician and can be reviewed by office personnel for completeness.

When assessing physical activity patterns of patients a number of self-reported methods can be used, ranging from very detailed questionnaires to shorter, more convenient methods. One of the most commonly used physical activity questionnaires is the seven-day physical activity recall (7-day PAR). While this method provides a very detailed assessment of physical activity, this questionnaire is rather lengthy (approximately 20 minutes to administer) and is done within an interview format. Thus, while a 7-day PAR may be very appropriate for research purposes, it is probably not practical for use within a primary care setting to assess the activity patterns of adults.

In a primary care setting, it is recommended that the physical activity assessment be short and concise so that the activity history can be reviewed by the physician during the limited time that he or she has with the patient. A sample of a questionnaire that meets these guidelines is presented in Figure 1. This questionnaire is similar to the questionnaire developed by Godin and Sheppard,[7] which has been shown to be reliable in adults.

Once regular activity behaviors are assessed, it is important to understand how this information can be used to promote a physically active lifestyle in patients. Currently, the **minimum** public health recommendation for physi-

FIGURE 1. Example of questionnaire to assess recent leisure-time fitness and sports activity history.

Instructions: Considering a typical 7-day period over the previous 3 months, how many times on average per week do you engage in at least 10 minutes of each of the categories of exercise listed below?	Episodes per Week	Average Minutes per Episode	Total Minutes per Week
Vigorous Activity (i.e., running/jogging, basketball game, cross-country skiing, inline skating, vigorous cycling, etc.)			
Moderate Activity (i.e., brisk walking, tennis, dancing, cycling for leisure, alpine skiing)			
Light Activity (i.e., stetching, yoga, easy walking, bowling, fishing)			

Adapted from Godin G and Sheppard RJ. A simple method to assess exercise behavior in the community. *Can J Appl Sport Sci.* 10: 141-146, 1985

How many days per week do you participate in moderate or vigorous intensity activity similar to brisk walking for at least 30 minutes per day?

☐ 0-1 days per week
☐ 2-3 days per week
☐ 4-5 days per week

When you are unable to be physically active, what is the most common reason that you are not physically active?

_____

Please list 3 to 5 moderate intensity activities that you enjoy.
1. _____
2. _____
3. _____
4. _____
5. _____

cal activity is 30 minutes of moderate intensity physical activity on most, preferably all, days of the week.[13] This is commonly interpreted as a minimum of 150 minutes of moderate-intensity physical activity per week. Thus, a quick review of the physical activity history will illustrate whether the patient is achieving this minimum goal and whether additional intervention is required. For example, a patient may indicate that he or she takes a 30 minute brisk walk 5 days per week, and in this case no intervention is needed other than encouraging the patient to continue this pattern of physical activity. However, a patient may indicate that he or she is "busy" all day, but this activity is in the form of "light" intensity activity. In this case, the physician should reinforce the current activity behaviors but attempt to intervene and encourage the patient to undertake additional activity that is at least "moderate" in intensity.

When using an assessment tool such as the one provided, it is important to understand not only how to assess physical activity, but also to understand how to provide meaningful information and feedback to patients that may impact their physical activity behaviors. For example, the advice provided to a patient who reports very little physical activity may need to be different than the advice provided to a moderately active patient that has some difficulty sustaining this level of physical activity on a regular basis. Moreover, querying the patient on common barriers may provide critical information related to a lack of physical activity, and may provide much-needed information for the physician to provide adequate advice to the patient. Basic guidance based on the brief assessment of physical activity is illustrated in Figure 1, and explained in greater detail below.

■ Developing an Activity Plan

When developing a physical activity plan for an adult, a number of factors should be taken into consideration, including information on the patient's activity history, his or her level of physical fitness, and whether the patient is normal weight, overweight, or obese. For example, an individual may report being physically active but may also be relatively unfit and overweight. Likewise, an individual may be physically fit and still be overweight. An example of how these factors can be used to determine an activity program for patients is illustrated in Figure 2.

In addition to considering the factors mentioned above, the most important factor to consider for the overweight, physically inactive patient is the reason for not engaging in regular physical activity. Developing an activity program will be effective only if the individual is able to minimize barriers and implement this activity program on a regular basis. Think of exercise as a medication. If a patient experiences side-effects that prohibit the use of one medication, the medication is discontinued and a different one is prescribed. Physical activity should be treated in the same manner. If an individual has barriers that prohibit him or her from implementing the planned activity program, it is important to review the plan and modify it in an appropriate manner to minimize the barriers. Strategies for overcoming common barriers to physical activity are addressed later in this chapter.

The most common method of designing an exercise prescription is to follow the F.I.T.T. principle. Based on this principle, the **F**requency, **I**ntensity, **T**ime (duration of the activity), and **T**ype of activity need to be taken into consideration for an exercise prescription to be complete, and it may be important to conduct an assessment of fitness or exercise tolerance prior to prescribing these exercise components. In addition, it is important to note

Figure 2. Physical Activity Intervention Model for Overweight/Obese Adults

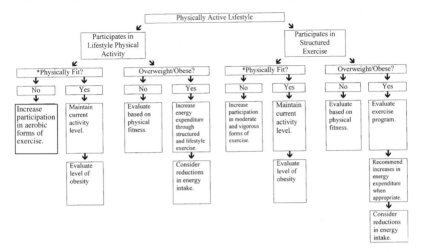

*Defined as at least in the moderate fitness category according to age and gender criteria.

that these components (frequency, intensity, time, and type of exercise) cannot be prescribed independently. For example, there is an inverse relationship between exercise intensity and exercise duration. As the intensity of the activity increases, the likelihood that the person will sustain the activity for a long duration is decreased. Conversely, a person will need to exercise for a much longer duration when the exercise intensity is low. When considering these factors, it is important to tailor the program to the needs of the individual patient. Activity programs should target a minimum of 150 minutes of moderate intensity activity per week (approximately 1000–1500 kcal/week), as this level of activity has been shown to be linked to improvements in morbidity and mortality. Once this level of activity is achieved, it may be beneficial to progressively increase above this level, as there is some evidence suggesting that approximately 250–300 minutes per week (approximately 2000–2500 kcal/wk) of activity is important for improving long-term weight loss.

Frequency of Activity

It has been shown that improvements in cardiorespiratory fitness can occur with 3–5 days of adequate intensity physical activity. However, current physical activity guidelines suggest that individuals should engage in moderate intensity physical activity "on most, preferably all, days of the week."[13] There are a number of reasons why overweight adults should engage in planned physical activity more often than 3 times per week. For example, for the purpose of body weight management, the greater the energy expenditure the greater the impact on body weight. In addition, planning activity into the daily routine may have a positive impact on adoption of regular physical activity behaviors. Thus, similar to other forms of medication that may be prescribed, patients should be encouraged to participate in adequate amounts of physical activity on a daily basis.

Intensity of the Activity

An important factor that needs to be taken into consideration is the intensity of the activity that is prescribed. There is some evidence that more vigorous activity may have a greater impact on health and fitness-related variables. However, individuals self-select activities that are of moderate intensity when given the option of choosing the type of activity they will perform. For most inactive adults, this would be the equivalent of brisk walking.

When prescribing the exercise intensity, it is common to prescribe the intensity based on the percentage of maximal heart rate, with the most accurate method of assessing maximal heart rate determined from a maximal graded exercise test. However, for relatively healthy, non-medicated adults, the maximal heart rate can be predicted using a simple equation (maximal heart rate = 220 − age). Regardless of whether the heart rate is measured or estimated, the exercise training intensity can be determined using a percentage of maximal heart rate or a percentage of maximal heart rate reserve. The computations for determining the appropriate exercise intensity and the recommendations for defining both moderate and vigorous exercise are shown in Table 1.

Even though prescribing exercise based on heart rate is commonly used, there may be factors that prohibit patients from actually monitoring their heart rate during exercise. For example, many individuals have a difficult time palpating their heart rate accurately, and this can lead to exercising at the incorrect intensity. Wearing a portable heart rate monitor is a potential solution. If this is too expensive for a patient, other methods of monitoring exercise intensity may need to be used. One such method is the Rating of Perceived Exertion. This technique requires that a patient rate their perceived effort based on a numeric scale, with the most common scale being the Borg 15-Point Category Scale.[1] On this scale, a rating of 6–7 corresponds to "very, very light," whereas a rating of 19–20 corresponds to "very, very hard." When prescribing exercise intensity that is of moderate intensity, a rating of 12–13 on this scale would be appropriate, with vigorous receiving a rating of 14–16. The use of perceived exertion has been shown to provide an accurate estimate of exercise intensity, and therefore may provide an alternative to using heart rate to monitor exercise intensity for most individuals. For best results it may be useful to walk individuals at a brisk pace within a hallway or corridor to anchor the feeling of moderate intensity for them.

Time (Duration of the Activity)

The duration of the activity is inversely related to exercise intensity and is typically based on a predetermined caloric expenditure. Therefore, an

TABLE 1. Computing Appropriate Exercise Intensity

Intensity Variable	Formula for Computing Exercise Intensity	Intensity Criteria	
		Moderate	Vigorous
Percentage of Maximal Heart Rate (%HRmax)	%HRmax = Maximal Heart Rate * desired %	55–69%	70–89%
Percentage of Maximal Heart Rate Reserve (%HRR)	% HRR = {(Maximal Heart Rate – Resting Heart Rate) * desired %} + Resting Heart Rate	40–59%	60–84%

Notes: 1. Maximal heart rate is determined from a maximal graded exercise test or can be estimated using 220—age.
2. Desired % is determined based on the exercise intensity criteria, and refers to either "moderate" or "vigorous."

individual who is exercising at a vigorous intensity will need to exercise for a shorter duration than someone who is exercising at a moderate intensity to elicit the same caloric expenditure. Assuming that most overweight adults will prefer to exercise at a moderate intensity when beginning an exercise program, the initial goal should be for patients to progressively increase to a minimum of 150 minutes of activity per week (30 minutes, 5 days per week). When progressing to this minimal level, encouraging participants to engage in activity bouts that are at least 10 minutes in duration would be appropriate. It has been shown that accumulating exercise in bouts of at least 10 minutes can improve cardiorespiratory fitness,[4,8,9] and this may be an effective strategy to implement with overweight adults. See Table 2 for an example of how to progress exercise to at least 30 minutes per day using multiple bouts that are at least 10 minutes in duration. Because there is some evidence that levels of exercise greater than the minimal public health recommendation of 150 minutes of exercise per week may be important for long-term weight loss,[9,11,15] it may be appropriate to eventually encourage greater amounts of exercise for patients when appropriate.

Type of Activity

Choosing an activity that is most appropriate for patients can be a significant challenge. There are many exercise programs and pieces of equipment that claim to provide the greatest benefit. This can have a significant impact on the patient's perception and choice of exercise. However, aside from the exercise providing adequate physiologic benefits, one of the most important factors is whether the individual enjoys the selected activity and has the skill to participate in it. A good activity to recommend for most individuals is walking. Walking requires very little skill, can be performed almost anywhere, does not require the use of equipment other than comfortable clothing and shoes, and allows the individual to self-select exercise intensity.

Other forms of exercise may also benefit overweight adults. These include resistance training, yoga, and flexibility exercises, which may be good

TABLE 2. Example of an Exercise Progression for Overweight Adults

Treatment Week	Intensity %HRmax	Intensity %HRR	RPE	Frequency (Days per Week)	Duration (Minutes per Day) Continuous	Duration (Minutes per Day) Intermittent	Total Exercise* (Minutes per Week)
1	55–69%	40–59%	12–13	5	10 min.	1 bout @ 10 min.	50
2	55–69%	40–59%	12–13	5	10 min.	1 bout @ 10 min.	50
3	55–69%	40–59%	12–13	5	10 min.	1 bout @ 10 min.	50
4	55–69%	40–59%	12–13	5	10 min.	1 bout @ 10 min.	50
5	55–69%	40–59%	12–13	5	20 min.	2 bout @ 10 min.	100
6	55–69%	40–59%	12–13	5	20 min.	2 bout @ 10 min.	100
7	55–69%	40–59%	12–13	5	20 min.	2 bout @ 10 min.	100
8	55–69%	40–59%	12–13	5	20 min.	2 bout @ 10 min.	100
9	55–69%	40–59%	12–13	5	30 min.	3 bout @ 10 min.	150
10	55–69%	40–59%	12–13	5	30 min.	3 bout @ 10 min.	150
11	55–69%	40–59%	12–13	5	30 min.	3 bout @ 10 min.	150
12	55–69%	40–59%	12–13	5	30 min.	3 bout @ 10 min.	150

%HRmax = percent of maximal heart rate, %HRR = percent of maximal heart rate reserve, RPE = rating of perceived exertion.
*Patient may progress above these levels over time if appropriate.

adjuncts to walking or other forms of aerobic exercise because they improve muscular strength and endurance, while improving joint range of motion. However, resistance and flexibility exercises may result in less energy expenditure than walking or other forms of aerobic exercise performed over the same period of time. Despite claims that resistance exercise can significantly increase resting energy expenditure, there is little evidence that this occurs during periods of significant weight loss. Thus, the benefits of resistance exercise may be to increase functional ability (getting out of a chair, carrying groceries, etc.) rather than through direct impact on body weight.

There has also been some evidence that lifestyle exercise may be an appropriate form of exercise for the purpose of weight loss.[2] Lifestyle exercise has been described as performing activities as part of daily life and may include things such as taking the stairs rather than the elevator, cutting the grass, cleaning the house, gardening, etc. However, this concept may be confusing for patients to understand, and may give them the perception that they are sufficiently physically active. Lifestyle activity for the purpose of weight loss should be promoted within the context of a physically active lifestyle that may include structured periods of exercise. An example of how these intervention strategies can be used for developing the appropriate activity programs for overweight adults is illustrated in Figure 2. Pedometers can be used to provide real time feedback on daily activity levels. These devices measure the number of steps taken, are relatively inexpensive, and are widely available. Individuals who have a daily step count of 3,000–6,000 are sedentary, from 7–10,000 moderately active, 11–15,000 very active. Individuals can set step goals that increase by 250 steps per week in an effort to increase their overall activity levels within the context of their usual activities.

Strategies for Overcoming Barriers to Physical Activity

It is clear that physical activity is an important component of a weight management program. However, many overweight individuals are not physically active. From a clinical perspective, it is not only important to recommend a certain amount (duration and intensity of activity) of activity to patients, but also to assist them in overcoming barriers to a more physically active lifestyle. The following are behavioral strategies for overcoming some of the commonly reported barriers to participation in physical activity.

Lack of Time. With many individuals attempting to juggle a number of commitments such as family, work, etc., it is not surprising that "lack of time" is one of the most commonly reported barriers to participation in regular physical activity. When "lack of time" is reported, it is important to suggest strategies that can be effective for overcoming this barrier. As suggested in recent public health guidelines, recommending the accumulation of activity throughout the day may be an effective alternative to traditional approaches to exercise. Studies have shown that exercising in bouts that are as short as 10 minutes in duration can impact on body weight, fitness, and coronary heart disease risk factors.[4,6,8,9] A patient could take a 10-minute walk during their lunch break, a 10-minute walk during their coffee break, and a 10-minute walk after dinner to accumulate 30 minutes of physical activity that day. This strategy has been shown to be an effective way to help an individuals begin to adopt a more active lifestyle that includes regular exercise.

Lack of Convenience. Another significant barrier commonly reported is that exercise is not convenient. This is most likely based on the perception a special facility such as a health club or gymnasium is required to exercise. This is a common misperception. It has been shown that self-directed exercise, home-based or performed in any manner that is convenient, improves adherence compared to exercise done under supervised conditions at specialized facilities.[10,14] Moreover, there is some evidence that home exercise equipment or living in close proximity to exercise and recreation facilities (e.g., parks, etc.) improves participation in exercise. Thus, identifying strategies that would allow participation in activity to be more convenient may be beneficial for patients who have difficulty adopting a more active lifestyle.

Lack of Enjoyment. Selecting activities that are enjoyable may be an extremely important factor in adoption and maintenance of a physically active lifestyle. For example, recommending that a patient join an aerobics class may not be effective if the individual does not enjoy that activity. When counseling patients about physical activity, it is important to ask about the types of activities that they enjoy. Recent studies examining the effectiveness of lifestyle approaches to physical activity have shown promise,[2,5] and this may be a result of individuals being counseled to identify activities that they enjoy, and then to identify strategies for incorporating these activities into their lifestyle.

Most of the information needed to develop a physical activity plan can be obtained from brief conversations with patients regarding their physical activity and exercise behaviors. When appropriate, a more extensive assessment may need to be performed. Recommendations for when this more extensive evaluation may be necessary are addressed below.

■ Clinical Exercise Testing Guidelines

Benefits of the Exercise Assessment

Performing an exercise assessment can provide valuable information to develop an appropriate exercise prescription for patients. The assessment can be as simple as administering a health history questionnaire such as the Physical Activity Readiness Questionnaire (PAR-Q) to performing a maximal graded exercise test. However, the quality of the information obtained is dependent on the type of assessment performed. The information obtained from a PAR-Q will provide general information about a patient's potential risk for exercise participation, whereas a graded exercise test provides information regarding specific responses to an exercise stimulus. There are also distinct cost and time differences between the various types of exercise assessments that need to be considered. Not all patients will need an extensive assessment before beginning an exercise program. How is it determined whether an exercise assessment should be performed, and if so, which one to choose?

Determining When to Conduct a Graded Exercise Test

When determining when an exercise test is indicated prior to a patient undertaking an exercise program, there are a number of factors that should be considered. These include the following:

- ✔ Are there risk factors present that may preclude or increase the risk of participation in an exercise program?
- ✔ Is there a medical history of cardiovascular disease, metabolic disorders, or other factors that may raise concerns over safety during exercise?
- ✔ Based on the medical history, is it appropriate for the patient to participate in unsupervised exercise?
- ✔ What is the mode and intensity of the exercise that will be performed?
- ✔ Does the fitness level of the participant appear to be compromised, and does this increase the risk that may be associated with exercise for the patient?

It is important to determine, based on the medical history, which participants may be at high risk for experiencing an adverse event while engaging in moderate to vigorous exercise. Persons classified as **low risk** would be men under the age of 45 and women under the age of 55 who do not currently experience any symptoms of cardiovascular disease and who have no more than one coronary artery disease risk factor. These risk factors include: family history of coronary artery disease, current or recent (within past 6 mos.), cigarette smoking, hypertension, hypercholesterolemia, impaired fasting glucose, obesity, and sedentary lifestyle. A **moderate risk** classification would include men $\geq$ 45 years of age, women $\geq$ 55 years of age, and anyone who has more than one coronary artery disease risk factor. **High risk** individuals are those currently experiencing signs or symptoms suggesting cardiovascular and pulmonary disease (pain in chest or neck, dizziness, or unusual fatigue with normal activities) or anyone with known pulmonary, cardiovascular, or metabolic disease.

Depending on the risk level of the patient, a graded exercise test may still not be warranted if the patient does not plan on participating in vigorous intensity activities. Many patients (especially those who are sedentary and/or overweight) will naturally self-select exercise intensities that are more moderate. However, it is important to differentiate between absolute and relative exercise intensities. A commonly used method of doing this is through the use of METs (metabolic equivalents). One MET is equal to the amount of energy expended during one minute of rest. Thus, an activity that is 3 METs would be equivalent to 3 times the energy expended at rest. Absolute moderate intensity activity is considered to be between 3 and 6 METs, whereas absolute vigorous intensity activity is anything greater than

6 METs. However, even moderate intensity activities such as walking may be considered vigorous for a highly inactive or unfit patient. For example, consider a patient with a low maximal capacity (e.g., 4 METs), who wishes to begin an exercise program and decides to start walking for 20 minutes at 3 mph on the local high school track. Even though this activity (~3.3 METs) is considered moderate intensity activity at absolute values, it actually requires 83% of the patient's maximal capacity to perform, which would classify it as a vigorous activity for this individual. Therefore, one of the main aims of the exercise assessment is to assess maximal capacity in individuals at moderate/high risk and/or for those who are extremely sedentary or unfit and determine exercise tolerance. Figure 3 provides a flow-chart for determining when an exercise test is necessary, and which assessment to perform on patients planing to engage in an exercise program.

Choosing the Appropriate Exercise Assessment

If it would be beneficial to obtain a measurement of cardiorespiratory fitness or exercise tolerance, there are a number of options to choose from. A summary of these options along with the potential benefits or limitations of each are summarized below.

When seeking an estimate of cardiorespiratory fitness in relatively healthy adults, it is possible to use a non-exercise prediction equation. One commonly used prediction equation is the Houston Non-Exercise Test. The Houston Non-Exercise Test estimates fitness using prediction equations that take into consideration a person's physical activity level, age, and body mass index or percent body fat (if available). Advantages of this test are that it appears to be reliable, does not require expensive equipment or staff, and is fairly easy to administer. However, this test provides no information regarding the cardiovascular response to an exercise stimulus, and will therefore provide no information on potential contraindications to exercise training that might otherwise go undetected.

When a functional test is desired, a submaximal protocol may be appropriate. Submaximal exercise tests can be performed using a variety of exercise modalities including treadmill, cycle ergometer, or a step test. An advantage of a submaximal exercise test is that it can be used to assess exercise tolerance across a spectrum of intensities without pushing patients to a maximal level. In addition, most submaximal exercise tests can be used to predict maximal fitness level within an acceptable tolerance of 10–15% of actual values. A disadvantage of a submaximal test is that it will not allow you to detect adverse responses to exercise that may occur near maximal effort.

Maximal graded exercise tests performed to volitional exhaustion may provide the most meaningful information related to the cardiovascular response to an exercise stimulus. A maximal test has greater sensitivity and specificity for determining whether cardiovascular abnormalities are present. Moreover, a maximal exercise test will provide very specific information relative to maximal heart rate, and this may be extremely valuable especially

FIGURE 3. Recommendations for Exercise Assessment Based on Risk Stratification

Risk Stratification	Exercise Intensity		Exercise Testing Recommations
Low Risk ↗ ↘	Moderate Intensity	↗	Submaximal Testing Not Required
		↘	Maximal Testing Not Required
	Vigorous Intensity	↗	Submaximal Testing Not Required
		↘	Maximal Testing Not Required
Moderate Risk ↗ ↘	Moderate Intensity	↗	Submaximal Testing Not Required
		↘	Maximal Testing Not Required
	Vigorous Intensity	↗	*Submaximal Testing without Physician Supervision
		↘	Maximal Testing with Physician Supervision
High Risk ↗ ↘	Moderate Intensity	↗	*Submaximal Testing with Physician Supervision
		↘	Maximal Testing with Physician Supervision
	Vigorous Intensity	↗	*Submaximal Testing with Physician Supervision
		↘	Maximal Testing with Physician Supervision

*The submaximal exercise test should be conducted so that it exceeds the exercise intensity that will be prescribed as part of the activity plan. In some situations, a maximal test may be more appropriate as it is more conclusive for ruling out coronary artery disease and determining adverse responses to exercise.

when determining an appropriate exercise intensity for patients with disease and patients taking medication that may affect the heart rate response during exercise. Despite these benefits, patients may find maximal tests uncomfortable, and there are data to suggest that overweight adults may not achieve a true maximal effort based on traditional physiologic criteria.

Detailed descriptions of commonly used graded exercise testing protocols as well as the descriptions and prediction equations used during submaximal exercise testing are described in detail in the American College of Sports Medicine's Guidelines for Exercise Testing and Prescription, 6th Edition.[1]

■ Summary

A physically active lifestyle that includes periods of regular physical activity is an important part of a weight management program. Exercise can also reduce morbidity and mortality rates from a variety of chronic diseases, and this appears to be independent of the effects on body weight. However, despite these benefits, many overweight adults are physically inactive and could benefit from increasing their participation in regular physical activity and exercise. Physicians and other health care professionals can address the importance of physical activity as part of regular visit with patients, and encourage the adoption of activity that results in a minimum of 150 minutes of activity per week. It is important for health care professionals to be sensitive to barriers that individuals are confronted with, and to assist patients with developing strategies to overcome these barriers.

References

1. American College of Sports Medicine: Guidelines for exercise testing and prescription. Philadelphia, PA, Lippincott, Williams and Wilkins, 2000.
2. Andersen RE, Wadden TA, Bartlett SJ, Zemel B, Verde TJ, Franckowiak SC: Effects of lifestyle activity vs structured aerobic exercise in obese women: a randomized trial. JAMA 281:335–340, 1999.
3. Barlow CE, Kohl III HW, Gibbons LW, Blair SN: Physical activity, mortality, and obesity. Int J Obes 19:S41–S44, 1995.
4. DeBusk RF, Stenestrand U, Sheehan M, Haskell WL: Training effects of long versus short bouts of exercise in healthy subjects. Am J Cardiol 65:1010–1013, 1990.
5. Dunn AL, Marcus BH, Kampert JB, Garcia ME, Kohl III HW, Blair SN: Comparison of lifestyle and structured interventions to increase physical activity and cardiorespiratory fitness. JAMA 281:327–334, 1999.
6. Ebisu Ebisu T: Splitting the distances of endurance training: on cardiovascular endurance and blood lipids. Jap J Phys Educ 30:37–43, 1985.
7. Godin G, Sheppard RJ: A simple method to assess exercise behavior in the community. Can J Appl Sport Sci 10: 141–146, 1985
8. Jakicic JM, Wing RR, Butler BA, Robertson RJ: Prescribing exercise in multiple short bouts versus one continuous bout: effects on adherence, cardiorespiratory fitness, and weight loss in overweight women. Int J Obes 19:893–901, 1995.
9. Jakicic JM, Winters C, Lang W, Wing RR: Effects of intermittent exercise and use of home exercise equipment on adherence, weight loss, and fitness in overweight women: a randomized trial. JAMA 282: 1554–1560, 1999.
10. King AC, Haskell WL, Taylor CB, Kraemer HC, DeBusk RF: Group- vs home-based exercise training in healthy older men and women. A community-based clinical trial. JAMA 266:1535–1542, 1991.
11. Klem ML, Wing RR, McGuire MT, Seagle HM, Hill JO: A descriptive study of individuals successful at long-term maintenance of substantial weight loss. Am J Clin Nutr 66:239–246, 1997.
12. Lee CD, Jackson AS, Blair SN: U.S. weight guidelines: is it also important to consider cardiorespiratory fitness? Int J Obes 22(suppl 2):S2–S7, 1998.
13. Pate RR, Pratt M, Blair SN, et al: Physical activity and public health. A recommendation from the Centers for Disease Control and Prevention and the American College of Sports Medicine. JAMA. 273:402–407, 1995.

14. Perri MG, Martin AD, Leermakers EA, Sears SF, Notelovitz M: Effects of group- versus home-based exercise in the treatment of obesity. J Consult Clin Psychol 65:278–285, 1997.
15. Schoeller DA, Shay K, Kushner RF: How much physical activity is needed to minimize weight gain in previously obese women? Am J Clin Nutr 66:551–556, 1997.
16. Wei M, Kampert JB, Barlow CE, et al: Relationship between low cardiorespiratory fitness and mortality in normal-weight, overweight, and obese men. JAMA 282: 1547–1553, 1999.

Chapter 13

David Heber, MD, PhD

Non-Prescription Weight-loss Products

In the last decade, the use of herbal and alternative medicines has increased, and the market for over-the-counter products for weight reduction is particularly strong. As the population becomes heavier, non-prescription products which promise quick and easy weight loss are attractive to the consumer. One reason for the appeal of alternative treatments is that professional assistance is not required for their use. For those who cannot afford to see a physician or other health care provider for weight-loss counseling, purchasing products over-the-counter represents a more accessible solution. For many others, these approaches may also be viewed as alternatives to failed attempts at weight loss using more conventional approaches. Without supervision, however, individuals who might be discouraged by previous failures are likely to combine approaches, or use these supplements at doses higher than what is recommended.

There are biologic rationales for the actions of the different alternative medical and herbal approaches to weight loss. Thermogenic aids such as ephedra and caffeine, synephrine, tea catechins, and chili pepper capsaicin are directed at increasing fat burning or metabolism during dieting. Many overweight individuals blame their weight on a "slow metabolism." Other supplements, such as *Garcinia cambogia*, claim to result in nutrient partitioning, so that dietary calories will be directed to muscle rather than fat. Still other approaches attempt to influence food intake and satiety through effects on noradrenergic, serotoninergic, or dopaminergic mechanisms. These include supplementary tyrosine, phenylalanine, and 5-hydroxytryptophan. A binding resin, chitosan, has been promoted as a "fat blocker" since it has been found to precipitate fat in solution in the laboratory.

■ Caffeine and Ephedrine

The most widely used herbal approaches for weight loss are dietary supplements that contain ephedra alkaloids (sometimes called *ma huang*). These are widely promoted and used as a means of weight loss by purportedly increasing energy expenditure. In light of recently reported adverse events related to use of these products, the Food and Drug Administration (FDA) has proposed limits on the dose and duration of their use.

Selling caffeine and ephedrine in herbal form for weight loss is a large industry. Caffeine in the herbal products is the same chemical contained in pharmaceutical caffeine. The scientific evidence in animals and humans supports a potential role for caffeine in weight reduction through increases in oxygen consumption and fat oxidation. Caffeine has a long history of safe use in food and has been used in headache preparations and to treat fatigue. The FDA approves caffeine for sale without a prescription for use as a stimulant by persons 12 years of age or older at a dose up to 200 mg every 3 hours (1600 mg/d) and as an ingredient in pain medications.

In a 3-month trial comparing ephedrine 25 mg tid and 50 mg tid with placebo, similar weight losses were observed in all groups with significantly more side effects (blood pressure elevation, pulse elevation, agitation, insommia, headache, weakness, palpitations, giddiness, euphoria, tremor and diarrhea) in the ephedrine 50 mg tid group compared to placebo.[1] There was more weight loss in the ephedrine groups, however, at the end of the first and second months, a difference that was lost by the end of the third month.[2]

In another study, a combination of 20 mg ephedrine with 200 mg caffeine given three times a day was studied in obese subjects randomized to ephedrine 20 mg tid, caffeine 200 mg tid, ephedrine 20 mg with caffeine 200 mg tid or placebo for a 24-week double blind trial. Weight loss with caffeine and ephedrine was greater than placebo from 8 weeks to the end of the trial. Ephedrine alone and caffeine alone were not different than placebo. The caffeine with ephedrine group lost 17.5% of their body weight in the 24-week trial. Side effects of tremor, insomnia, and dizziness reached the levels of placebo by 8 weeks, and blood pressure fell similarly in all four groups. After a two-week washout period at the end of the trial, headache and tiredness were more frequent in the group that had taken caffeine with ephedrine, and all subjects were given the opportunity to participate in an additional 24-week open-label trial using caffeine with ephedrine. Those subjects remaining on caffeine with ephedrine maintained their weight loss to the end of trial at week 50.[3] Seventy-five percent of the weight loss was explained by anorexia and 25% was explained by increased thermogenesis.[4]

Attempts have been made to explore the mechanisms by which ephedrine exerts its effects in humans. Although ephedrine stimulates brown adipose tissue in rodents, ephedrine-induced thermogenesis in humans takes place primarily in skeletal muscle, since humans have little brown adipose tissue.[5] Ephedrine has also been shown to decrease gastric emptying, which may contribute to its effect on food intake.[6]

Ephedrine and caffeine have each been sold for years without a prescription for the treatment of asthma and to combat drowsiness, respectively. Toxicity has not been a concern, even with recommended doses higher than that used in herbal products containing caffeine and ephedrine for weight loss. Ephedrine products sold without a prescription for the treatment of asthma have a recommended dosage up to 150 mg per day. Caffeine sold without a prescription has a recommended dose up to 1600 mg per day. The popular herbal products containing caffeine and ephedrine and taken for weight loss have dosage recommendations up to 100 mg of ephedrine equivalent per day as ephedra. The caffeine content of these herbal products containing caffeine and ephedrine varies but is less than 600 mg a day. The most popular and widely sold herbal product containing caffeine and ephedra contains only 240 mg of caffeine per day, less than 3 cups of coffee.

■ Green Tea Catechins

Green tea leaves are prepared by heating or steaming the leaves of *Camelia sinensis* soon after the leaves are picked, and this tea is widely consumed on a regular basis throughout Asia. Black tea is made by allowing the green tea leaves to auto-oxidize enzymatically, which leads to the conversion of a large percentage of green tea catechins to theaflavins. The catechins are a family of compounds, which includes epigallocatechin gallate (EGCG), considered to be the most potent antioxidant in the family. The catechins appear to be able to enhance sympathetic nervous system activity at the level of the fat-cell adrenoreceptor.

Since caffeine occurs naturally in green tea extract, it has been difficult to separate the effects of green tea from caffeine in humans. However, in a recent study by Dulloo et al,[7] subjects were given green tea extract capsules three times per day, providing a total of 150 mg caffeine and 375 mg total catechins of which 270 mg was EGCG. Subjects spent three 24-hour periods in an energy chamber during which they received the green tea extract, 150 mg of caffeine, or placebo. Energy expenditure was higher by 4.5% in the green tea period compared to placebo and 3.2% higher than when the same dose of caffeine was given alone. In addition, fat oxidation was increased. The net effect attributable to green tea could be estimated at approximately 80 calories/day. Clearly, it is difficult to demonstrate the effects of green tea catechins alone, but there is the possibility of a synergistic interaction with ephedrine independent of the caffeine content of green tea, which should be evaluated.

■ *Garcinia cambogia* (Hydroxycitric Acid)

Garcinia cambogia contains hydroxycitric acid (HCA) which is extracted from the rind of the brindall berry. HCA is one of 16 isomers of citric acid and the only one that inhibits citrate lyase, the enzyme that catalyzes the first step in fatty acid synthesis outside the mitochondrion.

A few clinical trials have evaluated the efficacy and safety of HCA. One trial evaluated a product containing both HCA from *Garcinia cambogia* and chromium picolinate. In a single-arm open-label trial of 8 weeks in 77 adults, 500 mg of *Garcinia cambogia* extract was combined with 100 micrograms of chromium picolinate and administered 3 times per day. A 5.5% weight loss was seen in women and 4.9% weight loss in men.[8] In another trial, 10 males acted as their own controls in a crossover trial evaluating energy expenditure and substrate oxidation. There was no difference in respiratory quotient, energy expenditure, glucose, insulin, glucagon, lactate, or beta-hydroxybutyrate at rest or during exercise.[9] Finally, in a trial which randomized 135 obese adults using a double-blind placebo-controlled design, HCA 1500 mg/day was administered daily for 12 weeks, and both groups were given a low-fat, high-fiber diet. In this trial, there was no significant difference in the weight loss observed in both groups.[10] HCA is also sold as an herbal supplement containing the calcium salt for which the dose is 3 gm/day as a treatment for obesity. In rodents, the sodium salt of HCA has been demonstrated to reduce food intake and body fat content with no change in body protein. It is unclear whether the insolubility of the calcium salt or a species difference between rodents and humans is responsible for the lack of efficacy in humans. Further trials with measures of bioavailability are needed to resolve this issue, but the presently available HCA herbal dietary supplements appear to have no effect on human obesity.

■ Chromium Picolinate

Chromium picolinate is a dietary supplement that has gained popularity for both weightlifters and people desiring weight loss.[11] It enhances the effectiveness of insulin and has been called "glucose-tolerance factor." In one randomized, double-blind design, the effect of 200 mcg/day of chromium as chromium picolinate compared to placebo which was administered to students of both sexes beginning a 12-week weight training class was examined. Although there was an increase in circumferences and a decrease in skin folds in all groups, the only significant difference seen was a greater increase in body weight in the females supplemented with chromium picolinate compared to the other three groups.[12] These findings were confirmed by Grant et al., who studied 43 obese women using 400 mcg/d of chromium. Women taking chromium picolinate gained weight unless engaged in exercise, which lowered weight and the insulin response to glucose.[13]

Pasman et al. compared 200 mcg/day chromium picolinate to fiber, caffeine, and 50 grams of carbohydrate in 33 obese subjects during a 16-month weight loss study, the first two months of which included a very-low-calorie diet. Chromium had no effect on body composition.[14] Walker et al. compared 200 mcg of chromium picolinate with placebo in 20 wrestlers over 14 weeks. There was no effect of chromium on body composition or performance.[15] Campbell et al. evaluated the effect of chromium picolinate 200 mcg/day in 18 men between 56 and 69 years of age during a resistance-training program.[16] Chromium had no effect on body composition or strength.

Toxicology testing in animals suggests that chromium supplements have a wide margin of safety,[17] but chromium picolinate does not alter body composition in humans, and as such is not helpful for the treatment of obesity.

■ Beta-hydroxy-beta-methylbutyrate (HMB)

Beta-hydroxy-beta-methylbutyrate (HMB) is a metabolite of leucine that is sold as a supplement to burn fat and build both strength and muscle tissue. Nissen et al. reported that HMB supplementation at 1.5 to 3 grams per day reduced muscle catabolism and increased fat-free mass during a weight-lifting program of 2–6 weeks' duration.[18] These effects were not seen, however, in trained athletes.[19] Although supplementation with HMB has been shown to be safe in studies lasting 3 to 8 weeks, it has not yet been tested for efficacy in the treatment of obesity.[20]

■ Soluble and Insoluble Dietary Fibers

It has been suggested that the increase in obesity in Western countries since 1900 may be related to changes in dietary fiber. The fiber associated with starchy foods has decreased while the fiber associated with fruits and vegetables has increased.[21] Efforts to evaluate the association of dietary fiber with body-weight regulation began in the 1980's. Guar gum, a water-soluble fiber, has been shown to reduce hunger and weight more effectively than water-insoluble bran-fiber in the absence of a prescribed diet.[22]

The relationship between obesity and fiber has also been evaluated epidemiologically. Using food-frequency questionnaires, obese men and women have been shown to have significantly more fat and less fiber in their diets than lean men and women.[23] Total fiber intake was higher in the lean than the obese group and the grams of fiber/1000 kcal was inversely related to BMI.[24]

The bulk of evidence suggests that dietary fiber decreases food intake and decreases hunger and water-soluble fiber may be more efficient than water-insoluble fiber. Dietary fiber supplements (5–40 gm/day) lead to small (1–3 kg) weight losses greater than placebo. Although the weight loss obtained with dietary fiber is less than the 5% of initial body weight felt to confer clinically significant health benefits, the safety of dietary fiber and its other potential benefits on cardiovascular risk factors recommend it for inclusion in weight-reduction diets.

■ Chitosan

Chitosan is acetylated chitin from the exoskeletons of crustaceans, such as shrimp. The product is designed to bind to intestinal lipids, including cholesterol and triglycerides, and has received a great deal of attention as a potential weight-loss aid working through a "fat blocker" mechanism. In public demonstrations, chitosan is mixed with corn oil in a glass of water. The precipitation of the oil/chitosan complex and clarification of the solution is used to demonstrate how fat malabsorption and weight loss in humans would result. Individuals are promised that they can eat the fatty foods they desire without gaining weight.

Two double-blind clinical trials have been performed to evaluate the effect of chitosan 1200–1600 mg orally twice a day. One trial included 51 obese women who were treated for 8 weeks and resulted in no reduction in weight.[25] The second trial included 34 overweight men and women who were treated for 28 days without any weight reduction relative to control.[26] There were no serious adverse events or changes in either trial, and no changes in fat-soluble vitamins or iron metabolism were seen. It would appear that chitosan has the potential for weight reduction by binding dietary fat but is not effective in the doses presently used in humans.

■ Summary

The opportunities for additional research in this area are plentiful. Unfortunately, there has been relatively limited funding by comparison to funding for research on pharmaceuticals. However, botanical dietary supplements often contain complex mixtures of phytochemicals that have additive or synergistic interactions. The metabolism of families of related compounds may be different than the metabolism of purified crystallized compounds. Herbal medicines in some cases may be simply less purified forms of single active ingredients but in other cases represent unique formulations of multiple related compounds that may have superior safety and efficacy compared to single ingredients.

While nonprescription medications may be useful adjuncts to a behavioral weight loss program for some patients, it is also important to note that these products have not been subjected to the same degree of safety and efficacy testing as are FDA-approved drugs. For most of these products the magnitude of weight loss is somewhat less than is seen with currently available pharmaceuticals (Chapter 14), and as noted under each product, these compounds are not entirely free of side effects. However, the cost and side-effect profiles of nonprescription medications are generally less than those for prescription medications. It is important to make sure that patients do not have unrealistic expectations of the weight loss that they might expect from using over-the-counter medications, and that they not lose sight of the important role that behavior change will play in any successful weight-control program. Finally, drawing from the clinical experience with fen-phen, for most patients benefits experienced from a weight-loss medication go away when the medication is stopped. This means that if either prescription or nonprescription medications are included in a weight-loss program, they will probably need to be continued for as long as the patient desires weight reduction. A clinician should discuss the need for long-term treatment as the patient embarks on a course of therapy with any weight loss medication.

Overweight and obesity are common problems affecting more than half of the population, yet obesity is stigmatized by society. It is not surprising that an effective weight-loss product containing compounds with a long history of safe nonprescription use would be embraced enthusiastically by the public. Traditional herbal medicines may have more acceptance than prescription drugs in many cultures with emerging epidemics of obesity. A large number of ethnobotanical studies have found herbal treatments for diabetes, and similar surveys, termed bioprospecting, for obesity treatments may be productive in the future.

References

1. Pasquali R, Baraldi G, Cesari MP, et al: A controlled trial using ephedrine in the treatment of obesity. Int J Obes 9:93-8, 1985.
2. Pasquali R, Cesari MP, Besteghi L, Melchionda N, Balestra V: Thermogenic agents in the treatment of human obesity: preliminary results. Int J Obes 11:23-6, 1987.
3. Toubro S, Astrup A, Breum L, Quaade F: The acute and chronic effects of ephedrine/caffeine mixtures on energy expenditure and glucose metabolism in humans. Int J Obes Relat Metab Disord 17 Suppl 3:S73-7; discussion S82, 1993.
4. Astrup A, Toubro S, Christensen NJ, Quaade F: Pharmacology of thermogenic drugs. Am J Clin Nutr 55:246S-248S, 1992.
5. Astrup A: Thermogenesis in human brown adipose tissue and skeletal muscle induced by sympathomimetic stimulation. Acta Endocrinol Suppl 278:1-32, 1986.
6. Jonderko K, Kucio C: Effect of anti-obesity drugs promoting energy expenditure, yohimbine and ephedrine, on gastric emptying in obese patients. Aliment Pharmacol Ther 5:413-8, 1991.
7. Dulloo AG, Seydoux J, Girardier L, Chantre P, Vandermander J: Green tea and thermogenesis: interactions between catechin-polyphenols, caffeine and sympathetic activity. Int J Obes Relat Metab Disord 24:252-8, 2000.
8. Badmaev V, Majeed M: Open field, physician-controlled clinical evaluation of botanical weight loss formula citrin. Nutracon: Nutraceuticals, dietary supplements and functional foods. Las Vegas, Nevada, 1995.
9. Kriketos AD, Thompson HR, Greene H, Hill JO: Hydroxycitric acid does not affect energy expenditure and substrate oxidation in adult males in a post-absorptive state. Int J Obes Relat Metab Disord 23:867-73, 1999.
10. Heymsfield SB, Allison DB, Vasselli JR, Pietrobelli A, Greenfield D, Nunez C: Garcinia cambogia (hydroxycitric acid) as a potential antiobesity agent: a randomized controlled trial. JAMA 280:1596-600, 1998.
11. Porter DJ, Raymond LW, Anastasio GD: Chromium: friend or foe? Arch Fam Med 8:386-90, 1999.
12. Hasten DL, Rome EP, Franks BD, Hegsted M: Effects of chromium picolinate on beginning weight training students. Int J Sport Nutr 2:343-50, 1992.
13. Grant KE, Chandler RM, Castle AL, Ivy JL: Chromium and exercise training: effect on obese women. Med Sci Sports Exerc 29:992-8, 1997.
14. Pasman WJ, Westerterp-Plantenga MS, Saris WH: The effectiveness of long-term supplementation of carbohydrate, chromium, fibre and caffeine on weight maintenance. Int J Obes Relat Metab Disord 21:1143-5, 1997.
15. Walker LS, Bemben MG, Bemben DA, Knehans AW: Chromium picolinate effects on body composition and muscular performance in wrestlers. Med Sci Sports Exerc 30:1730-7, 1998.
16. Campbell WW, Joseph LJ, Davey SL, Cyr-Campbell D, Anderson RA, Evans WJ: Effects of resistance training and chromium picolinate on body composition and skeletal muscle in older men. J Appl Physiol 86:29-39, 1999.
17. Anderson RA, Bryden NA, Polansky MM: Lack of toxicity of chromium chloride and chromium picolinate in rats. J Am Coll Nutr 16:273-9, 1997.
18. Nissen S, Sharp R, Ray M, et al: Effect of leucine metabolite beta-hydroxy-beta-methylbutyrate on muscle metabolism during resistance-exercise training. J Appl Physiol 81:2095-104, 1996.

19. Van Itallie TB: Dietary fiber and obesity. Am J Clin Nutr 31:S43-52, 1978.
20. Krotkiewski M: Effect of guar gum on body-weight, hunger ratings and metabolism in obese subjects. Br J Nutr 52:97-105, 1984.
21. Kreider RB, Ferreira M, Wilson M, Almada AL: Effects of calcium beta-hydroxy-beta-methylbutyrate (HMB) supplementation during resistance-training on markers of catabolism, body composition and strength. Int J Sports Med 20:503-9, 1999.
22. Nissen S, Sharp RL, Panton L, Vukovich M, Trappe S, Fuller JC: Beta-hydroxy-beta-methylbutyrate (HMB) supplementation in humans is safe and may decrease cardiovascular risk factors. J Nutr 130:1937-45, 2000.
23. Miller WC, Niederpruem MG, Wallace JP, Lindeman AK: Dietary fat, sugar, and fiber predict body fat content. J Am Diet Assoc 94:612-5, 1994.
24. Alfieri MA, Pomerleau J, Grace DM, Anderson L: Fiber intake of normal weight, moderately obese and severely obese subjects. Obes Res 3:541-7, 1995.
25. Wuolijoki E, Hirvela T, Ylitalo P: Decrease in serum LDL cholesterol with microcrystalline chitosan. Methods Find Exp Clin Pharmacol 21:357-61, 1999.
26. Pittler MH, Abbot NC, Harkness EF, Ernst E: Randomized, double-blind trial of chitosan for body weight reduction. Eur J Clin Nutr 53:379-81, 1999.

Chapter 14

Robert Kushner, MD

Pharmacologic Therapy

Use of drugs as an adjunct to lifestyle approaches is a familiar and time-honored concept. For instance, cholesterol-lowering agents, antihypertensives and antidiabetic drugs are commonly prescribed for patients assessed at high risk and for whom dietary and physical activity therapy has not been successful. However, when it comes to prescribing anti-obesity medications, there is often more reservation and skepticism. This misgiving stems, in part, from the past use of amphetamine-derived addictive stimulant medications and the disastrous results of the fen-phen period. Moreover, many physicians are still wary of prescribing anorexiants due to having very little to no experience in how to use them, and from a general lack of knowledge about obesity itself. Since 1997, two anti-obesity medications, sibutramine (Meridia) and orlistat (Xenical), have been approved by the FDA for long-term use. This chapter will review the use of pharmacotherapy, the available agents, and anticipated results of treatment.

■ Overview

There are several potential targets of pharmacologic therapy for obesity, all based on the concept of producing a sustained negative energy (calorie) balance. The earliest and most thoroughly explored treatment has been suppression of appetite via centrally active medications that alter monoamine neurotransmitters. A second strategy is to reduce the absorption of selective macronutrients from the gastrointestinal tract, such as fat. These two mechanisms form the basis for all currently prescribed antiobesity agents. Over the counter (OTC) agents include drugs and herbs that diminish taste (benzocaine), produce gastric fullness and satiety (fiber-containing substances), and reduce appetite (phenylpropanolamine, ephedra). These approaches are reviewed in chapter 13. Further understanding of appetite regulation and energy metabolism will bring new and exciting pharmacological agents to the market over the next 10 years. Promising areas of research include selective dopaminergic agents that alter appetite; administration of synthetic analogues or inhibitors of several neuropeptides, including leptin, neuropeptide Y (NPY), and melanocortin, which may both reduce caloric intake and increase energy expenditure; agents that stimulate thermogenesis such as selective beta-3 adrenergic receptor agonists; and drugs that may interfere with energy utilization or nutrient partitioning. Several recent articles provide a comprehensive review of the current and future pharmacological treatment of obesity.[1-3]

One of the fundamental concepts about any pharmacological approach to obesity is the importance of the drug-behavior interaction. Whether the medication acts centrally to suppress appetite or peripherally to block the absorption of fat, patients must deliberately and consciously alter their behavior for weight loss to occur. In other words, for all antiobesity drugs, the pharmacological action must be translated into behavior change. For anorexiants, a reduced sense of hunger and/or increased satiety must be translated into choosing smaller, healthier meals and reduced snacking. Failure to sense and act upon these inhibitory internal signals will result in modest or no weight loss. Similarly, if a patient takes an intestinal fat blocking agent and does not limit the consumption of dietary fat to 30% or less, he or she will discontinue the medication due to intolerable side effects. Likewise, if this same patient increases the consumption of nonfat calories (protein, carbohydrate, and alcohol) to avoid any side effects, he or she may actually gain weight despite 100% compliance with the medication. Furthermore, failure to incorporate physical activity as part of the lifestyle change will seriously hinder maintenance of the initial weight loss. Thus, there is a bi-directional, mutually beneficial relationship between antiobesity drugs and lifestyle management, each therapy enhancing the efficacy of the other. It is for this reason that all antiobesity medications should be used as adjuncts to, and not substitutes for, lifestyle change.

■ Centrally Acting Anorexiant Medications

Appetite-suppressing drugs, or anorexiants, effect *satiation*—the processes involved in the termination of a meal, *satiety*—the absence of hunger after eating, and *hunger*—a biological sensation that initiates eating. By increasing satiation and satiety and decreasing hunger, these agents help patients reduce caloric intake while providing a greater sense of control, more contentment with food intake, and with reduced feelings of deprivation. The target site for the actions of anorexiants is the ventromedial and lateral hypothalamic regions in the central nervous system. Their biological effect on appetite regulation is produced by variably augmenting the neurotransmission of three monoamines: norepinephrine, serotonin (5-hydroxytryptamine, 5-HT), and to a lesser degree, dopamine. The classical sympathomimetic adrenergic agents function by either stimulating norepinephrine release or blocking its reuptake. In contrast, the two serotonergic agents that were withdrawn from the U.S. market in September 1997 were selective for stimulating serotonin release and blocking its reuptake. A third type of anorexiant drug, sibutramine, functions as a serotonin and norepinephrine reuptake inhibitor (SNRI). The specific mechanisms of action of these drugs, brand names, and dosing is shown in Table 1. Drugs approved for long-term use by the FDA are shown in Table 2.

With the exception of sibutramine, all of the anorexiant drugs that are marketed for the treatment of obesity are related chemically and pharmacologically to amphetamine. By modifying either the aliphatic side chain or

TABLE 1. Comparison of Antiobesity Agents

System	Generic name	Brand name	Mechanism	Dosage regimen	DEA schedule
Centrally Acting Adrenergic	benzphetamine	Didrex	Stimulates NE release	25mg to 50mg qd - tid	III
	phendimetrazine	Prelu-2 Bontril Plegine	Stimulates NE release	105mg SR qd	III
	diethylproprion	Tenuate	Stimulates NE release	25mg tid or 75mg SR qd	IV
	mazindol	Mazonor Sanorex	Blocks NE reuptake	1mg tid 1mg q d	IV
	phentermine	Adipex-P Fastin Ionamin	Stimulates NE release	37.5mg qd 30mg qd 15mg or 30mg qd	IV
	phenylpropa-nolamine	Acutrim Dexatrim Prolamine	Alpha-1 agonist	75mg SR qd 25mg tid or 75mg SR 37.5mg qd	OTC
Centrally Acting Serotonergic	fenfluramine	Pondimin	Stimulates 5-HT release	20mg tid	Removed from the market Sept, 1997
	dexfenfluramine	Redux	Stimulates 5-HT release	15mg BID	Removed from the market Sept, 1997
Centrally Acting Adrenergic and Serotonergic	sibutramine	Meridia	Serotonin and norepinephrine reuptake inhibitor (SNRI)	5, 10, 15mg qd	IV
Lipase Inhibitor	orlistat	Xenical	Gastric and pancreatic lipase inhibitor	120mg tid	Not scheduled

aromatic ring, the side effects of CNS excitation, euphoria, and chemical dependency are lessened. Prior to the early 1970's, more than 200 controlled short-term (1 to 3 month) studies were conducted demonstrating that these anorexiant agents resulted in an average weight loss of approximately one-half pound per week more than placebo. However, patients quickly regained weight once the medications were discontinued leading to the erroneous conclusion that drug therapy had no role in the treatment of obesity. In addition, their misuse and potentially addictive properties led the Drug Enforce-

TABLE 2. Weight Loss Drugs Approved for Long-Term Use*

Drug	Dose	Action	Adverse Effects
Sibutramine (Meridia)	5, 10, 15 mg (10mg po qd to start, may be increased to 15mg or decreased to 5 mg)	norepinephrine, dopamine, and serotonin reuptake inhibitor	increase in heart rate and blood pressure
Orlistat (Xenical)	120 mg (120 mg po tid before meals)	inhibits pancreatic lipase, decreases fat absorption	decrease in absorption of fat-soluble vitamins; soft stools and anal leakage

*Ephedrine and caffeine, mazindol, fluoxetine, and phentermine have also been tested for weight loss, but are not approved for long-term use.

Source: Adapted from the Practical Guide to the Identification, Evaluation, and Treatment of Overweight and Obesity in Adults (preprint). National Institutes of Health and the North American Association for the Study of Obesity, Bethesda, MD, September, 1998.

ment Agency (DEA) to schedule them as controlled substances. According to the Physicians Desk Reference, these older anorexiants are approved for short-term monotherapy management of exogenous obesity.

A reconsideration of drug therapy for obesity was primarily prompted by Weintraub et al. in the early 1980's. Reasoning that obesity is a chronic disease similar to diabetes or hypertension, long-term use of medications should be considered for a sustained control of body weight. Weintraub also applied a principle routinely used in the treatment of other diseases, that of combined drug administration. By prescribing two medications with different mechanisms of action and used in smaller amounts, one could achieve an efficacy equivalent to or greater than a high dose of a single agent and with fewer adverse effects. Thus, a long-term, prospective, randomized, double-blind trial was designed comparing the combined use of an adrenergic agent (phentermine) and a selective serotonergic agent (fenfluramine) compared to placebo in 121 patients with obesity.[4] During the first 6 months of the trial, those on combination therapy lost significantly more weight than those on placebo, 15.9% of initial weight versus 4.9%. For those subjects who completed the study, weight tended to be maintained or increase slightly for the duration of the 3.5 years of treatment. The landmark study demonstrated the feasibility and efficacy of long-term pharmacotherapy for obesity.

Based on Weintraub's initial observations, the combined off label use of phentermine and fenfluramine (dubbed fen-phen by the general public) was widely prescribed across the country. Dexfenfluramine, the active d-isomer of fenfluramine, was approved for use in the U.S. in 1996, the first new anti-obesity medication approved since 1973. Along with fen-phen, Redux™ was used by millions of overweight and obese individuals in the U.S. between 1994 and 1997. These medications resulted in an average weight loss of 10–17% in one year. The two serotonergic agents, fenfluramine and dexfenfluramine, were known to be associated with the potentially serious side effect of primary pulmonary hypertension (PPH). The International Primary Pulmonary Hypertension Study (IPPHS), an epidemiological case-control study that looked at the relationship between PPH and anorexiants, concluded that the risk of PPH in persons exposed to these drugs for three or more months was approximately 23 times higher than in nonusers. Multiple cases of PPH have been reported in patients who were exposed to these medications.

■ Valvular Heart Disease

The eventual withdrawal of fenfluramine and dexfenfluramine from the marketplace in September 1997 was not brought about by the increased risk for PPH but by an other unexpected complication. In July 1997, the Mayo Clinic reported on 24 patients who developed predominately left-sided valvular heart disease resulting from the use of these medications.[5] Excised valves were found to have features characteristic of those described in the carcinoid syndrome. This information immediately prompted the FDA to collect and analyze echocardiographic prevalence data from five separate surveys performed on patients treated with fen-phen or Redux™. Using a valvulopathy case definition of lesions $\geq$ mild aortic regurgitation (AR) and/or $\geq$ moderate mitral regurgitation (MR), abnormal echocardiograms were found in 30% to 38% of patients. Based on this preliminary survey information and the millions of Americans projected to have taken these medications nationwide, the FDA requested the voluntary withdrawal of fenfluramine and dexfenfluramine from the U.S. market. The manufacturers subsequently complied with the request on September 15, 1997.

Although the cause for the increased incidence of aortic regurgitation and mitral insufficiency remains unknown, multiple case-controlled and prospective studies suggest that the incidence is lower than reported previously (9% to 23%), is greater for AR than MR, and is related to duration of exposure ($\geq$ 3 to 4 months).[6] The new ACC/AHA Practice Guidelines recommend that all patients with a history of fenfluramine or dexfenfluramine use undergo a careful history and thorough physical examination, reserving use of 2-D and Doppler echocardiography for patients with symptoms, cardiac murmurs, or other signs of cardiac involvement.[7] Evidence linking phentermine use alone to the valvulopathy was not convincing. This drug remains as an approved anorexiant agent. However, its package insert now includes a warning stating that the possibility of an association between valvular heart disease and phentermine alone cannot be ruled out.

■ Sibutramine (Meridia)

Sibutramine (Meridia™) was approved in the U.S. in 1997. Unlike all previous anorexiant agents, sibutramine is not chemically related to amphetamine and functions as a dual serotonin and norepinephrine reuptake inhibitor. The drug's appetite-suppressing effect was serendipitously discovered during early trials as an antidepressant. Sibutramine produces a dose-related weight loss when given in the range of 5 to 30 mg daily. In a 24-week double-blind, placebo-controlled study by Bray et al, patients taking 10 mg and 15 mg daily of sibutramine (the recommended dosages for clinical use) lost on average 6.1% and 7.4% weight, respectively, compared to 1.2% for placebo.[8] The longest published use of sibutramine comes from the STORM (Sibutramine Trial of Obesity Reduction and Maintenance) Study Group.[9] In this study, all patients were prescribed sibutramine 10 mg daily (open label) along with a calorie control diet and exercise for the first 6 months. Patients achieving at least a 5% weight loss were then randomized to continue sibutramine or switched to a placebo (double-blind) for 18 additional months. Of the 499 patients who completed the first 6 months (18% withdraw before 6 months), 94% lost at least 5% weight and entered the second phase of the trial. Fifty-eight percent of the sibutramine group and 50% of the placebo group completed the study. At 24 months, mean weight loss was 22.5 pounds for the sibutramine group compared to 10.3 pounds for the placebo group. Approximately one-half of the sibutramine drop-out rate was due to adverse events. These trials have also demonstrated beneficial changes in waist and hip circumference, serum lipids, uric acid, and glycemic control.

Sibutramine has also been demonstrated to be useful in a study that employed a "stepped care approach" to obesity.[10] In this trial, patients were initially treated with a very-low-calorie diet (VLCD) for 4 weeks. Patients who lost at least 6 kg were then randomized to either sibutramine 10 mg or placebo for 12 months. In this two-stage treatment, patients lost approximately 7% body weight with the VLCD. Those randomized to sibutramine lost another 5.4% over the subsequent year compared to gaining back 0.5% weight on placebo. Thus, by combining two modalities—a VLCD followed by pharmacotherapy—a greater absolute weight loss is achieved. This treatment regimen is particularly useful to consider for patients with moderate to severe obesity, uncontrolled diabetes, fluid overload, or severe hypertriglyceridemia.

Sibutramine does not appear to adversely affect cardiac valve function or cause PPH. An echocardiographic study has shown no increased incidence of left-sided valvulopathy after a mean of 7.6 months of treatment. The most commonly reported adverse events are headache, dry mouth, insomnia, and constipation. In addition to probing for these side effects, patients taking this medication require periodic monitoring of blood pressure and heart rate. The use of 10–15 mg of sibutramine daily has been shown to cause a mean increase in heart rate of 3–6 beats/min and an average elevation in diastolic blood pressure of less than 4 mm Hg. Some patients may manifest greater elevations requiring a reduction in dosage or discontinuation of the medication entirely. Treatment typically begins with 10 mg once daily with patients seen again within one month. At that time a decision is made to either continue the medication, increase the dose to 15 mg if the drug is well-tolerated but anticipated affects on appetite and weight have not occurred, discontinue, or reduce the dosage to 5 mg if side effects occur. The medication can be given to patients with a history of hypertension as long as it is controlled. These effects are consistent with the mode of action of sibutramine as a SNRI. Sibutramine should not be used in patients with a history of CAD, arrhythmia, uncontrolled hypertension, or stroke. The drug is contraindicated in patients receiving monoamine oxidase inhibitors (MAOIs) and with other centrally active appetite suppressant agents. Caution is advised if the patient is also taking another serotonergic agent, such as one of the antidepressant SSRI's, venlafaxine (a SNRI), or a drugs that inhibit cytochrome P450(3A4), such as ketoconazole and erythromycin. Current studies by the manufacturer are addressing the safety and efficacy of a 20-mg dosage and the response to dose escalation.

■ Orlistat (Xenical)

The newest anti-obesity medication is orlistat (Xenical™), approved in the U.S. in 1999. Orlistat is the first non-systemic antiobesity drug that acts entirely in the gastrointestinal tract. As a pentaenoic acid ester, orlistat forms a covalent bond with the active serine residue site of gastric and pancreatic lipases, inhibiting their activity and preventing absorption of about 30% of dietary fat. Weight loss occurs as a consequence of two factors: the reduced absorption of dietary fat calories and the drug-induced adverse effects that promote dietary change. If one consumes a 2000 calorie 30% fat diet, orlistat would block the absorption of 22 grams of fat, or 200 calories daily. Over a month, this would lead to a calorie deficit of 6000 calories—equivalent to just under 2 lb of weight loss. The second therapeutic factor leading to weight loss is the negative reinforcement produced when the patient consumes a high fat meal, that of uncomfortable and often embarrassing GI side effects. When used as prescribed, orlistat can be beneficial for patients unable to control their weight with lifestyle management alone.

Several randomized placebo-controlled trials of one to two years duration have demonstrated the efficacy of orlistat as an antiobesity agent. Two large placebo-controlled trials tested the effects of orlistat 120 mg tid or placebo in addition to a low-calorie diet for one year, followed by a second year on the drug or placebo.[11,12] Both studies came to similar conclusions. On average, subjects on orlistat lost 10% of their weight at one year compared to a 6% weight loss with placebo. In the second year, patients who stayed on the drug regained 1.5 to 3 kg, compared to a 4 to 6 kg regain in patients switched to placebo. Improvements in total cholesterol, LDL-cholesterol, blood pressure, glucose, and insulin levels were also noted. A unique feature of orlistat is its independent effect on serum lipids. Since orlistat inhibits absorption of dietary fat, it can also be considered a pharmacologic lipid-lowering agent. In another study of obese patients with type-2 diabetes treated with oral sulfonylureas, the addition of orlistat resulted in significant improvements in plasma fasting glucose, HbA1c, lipid levels, and dosage reductions in oral sulfonylurea medication compared to placebo.[13] At the time of this writing, Hoffman-La Roche, manufacturers of Xenical, has submitted an application to the FDA to add the new indication for improvement of glycemic control in overweight or obese patients with type-2 diabetes when used in combination with other diabetes treatments.

The most significant feature determining patient compliance is the drug's adverse effects. All patients will notice oil in their stool, which is manageable if they control the amount of fat in their diet. However, 20 to 40% of patients taking orlistat will have a major GI side effect, such as increased defecation, flatulence with discharge, oily spotting and evacuation, fecal urgency, or fecal incontinence. For this reason, patients must be informed of how to properly take the medication and the importance of following a fat-reduced diet. The most significant safety concern regarding the medication is the malabsorption of lipid-soluble nutrients, such as the fat-soluble vitamins A, D, E, and K, beta-carotene, and other carotenoids. Plasma levels of these nutrients decreased more in the orlistat-treated groups compared to placebo; however, values stayed within reference ranges. Nonetheless, the manufacturer recommends that all patients take a daily multivitamin supplement containing fat-soluble vitamins and beta-carotene at least two hours before or after the administration of orlistat, such as at bedtime. The usual dosage is one 120 mg capsule tid with each fat-containing meal. Patients can take the medication during the meal or up to one hour afterward.

One additional caveat regarding orlistat use needs to be mentioned. There are four sources of calories in the diet: fat, carbohydrate, protein, and alcohol. Orlistat partially blocks the absorption of only one of these sources. If the patient increases the consumption of non-fat foods as an alternative to reducing fat in the diet, they may actually increase total caloric intake and gain weight despite being taking the medication. Thus, attention to the whole diet, including reduction of total calories, must be reinforced for the medication to be effective.

■ When to Start Pharmacotherapy

According to the package insert for both sibutramine and orlistat, the drugs are indicated for obesity management including weight loss and weight maintenance when used in conjunction with a reduced-calorie diet. Orlistat is also indicated to reduce the risk for weight regain after prior weight loss. Using the BMI categorization for obesity, both agents are indicated for individuals with a BMI of $\geq$ 30 or $\geq$ 27 in the presence of other risk factors. Beyond these global indications, the physician will want to make the decision to initiate pharmacotherapy based on the patient's medical risks, their inability to lose weight by lifestyle counseling alone, their understanding of how the drug works, and continued commitment to receive counseling and monitoring.

■ When to Stop Pharmacotherapy

Many patients who come to your office inquiring about a medication to help them lose weight want to use the medication for a short period of time to get a head start on a weight loss program. However, the clinical experience with fen-phen suggests that the benefits that come from using a weight loss medication tend to go away as soon as the medication is stopped. It is important that you discuss the potential need for long-term treatment for obesity when you discuss the role of weight loss medications with your patients. Prescribing weight loss medications for short time periods can reinforce a bias that many patients have that once they lose weight, their weight will stay at that new level without further attention. A more realistic view is that obesity is a chronic metabolic disorder, which in many people tends to progress as they age much like hypertension, hyperlipidemia, or diabetes. In this view, medications used as an adjunct to a behavioral weight loss program will need to be taken as long as the patient wants to reduce weight. While some patients may choose to use medications intermittently during periods when they are having difficulty adhering to their usual behavioral plan (holidays, winter, periods of stress), this approach has not been studied and is not the typical approach. It may be that weight loss medications can be tapered or stopped after several years of use, but it seems more likely the indications that prompted the use of the medications in the first place will remain for the rest of the patient's life.

References

1. Kordik CP, Reitz AB: Pharmacological treatment of obesity: Therapeutic strategies. J Medicinal Chem 42:181-201, 1999.
2. Bray GA, Greenway FL: Current and potential drugs for treatment of obesity. Endocrine Rev 20:805-875, 1999.
3. Collins P, Williams G: Drug treatment of obesity: from past failures to future successes? Br J Clin Pharmacol 51:13-25, 2001.
4. Weintraub M: Long-term weight control: the national heart, lung, and blood institute funded multidimodal intervention study. Clin Pharm and Ther 51:581-646, 1992.
5. Connolly HM, Crary JL, McGoon MD, Hensrud DD, et al: Valvular heart disease associated with fenfluramine-phentermine. N Engl J Med 337:581-588, 1997.
6. Gardin JM, Schumacher D, Constantine G, Davis KD, Leung C, Reid CL: Valvular abnormalities and cardiovascular status following exposure to dexfenfluramine or phentermine/fenfluramine. JAMA 283:1703-1709, 2000.
7. American College of Cardiology/American Heart Association : Guidelines for the management of patients with valvular heart disease. Circulation 98:1949-1984, 1998.
8. Bray GA, Blackburn GL, Ferguson JM, Greenway FL, et al: Sibutramine produces dose-related weight loss. Obesity Res 7:189-198, 1999.
9. James WPT, Finer N, Hilsted J, Kopelman P, et al: Effect of sibutramine on weight maintenance after weight loss: A randomized trial. Lancet 356:2119-2125, 2000.
10. Apfelbaum M, Vague P, Ziegler O, Hanotin C, Thomas F, Leutenegger E: Long-term maintenance of weight loss after a very-low-calorie diet: A randomized blinded trial of the efficacy and tolerability of sibutramine. Am J Med 106:179-184, 1999.

11. Davidson MH, Hauptman J, DiGirolamo M, Foreyt JP, et al. Weight control and risk factor reduction in obese subjects treated for 2 years with orlistat. A randomized controlled trial. JAMA 1999;281:235-242.

12. Sjostrom L, Rissanen A, Anderson T, Boldrin M, et al. Randomized placebo-controlled trial of orlistat for weight loss and prevention of weight regain in obese patients. Lancet 1998;352:167-172.

13. Hollander PA, Elbein SC, Hirsch IB, Kelley D, et al. Role of orlistat in the treatment of obese patients with type-2 diabetes. Diabetes Care 1998;21:1288-1294.

Chapter 15
Daniel H. Bessesen, MD

Ethical Considerations in the Use of Medications in the Treatment of Overweight and Obese Individuals

The withdrawal of fenfluramine and dexfenfluramine from the market left questions and concerns about the appropriateness of prescribing weight-loss medications. The realization that 10-30% of those who received these drugs may have developed valvular heart disease as a complication of therapy raised important ethical concerns in the minds of many who had reluctantly prescribed these medications under pressure from their patients. However, it is hard to ignore the experience that many of us had with patients who lost weight on these medications and whose health and quality of life improved a great deal with that weight loss. Was it wrong to prescribe these medications? Given the risks and benefits of the medications available today, should weight-loss medications be prescribed again? What values and principles should guide these decisions?

Despite the rising prevalence of obesity and its associated health problems, many primary care providers remain uncomfortable providing medications for obese individuals because of concerns that the risks outweigh potential benefits. In this environment a more formal consideration of the ethical issues raised by the use of weight loss medications may be useful. It is important not to overreact to the problems with fenfluramine and dexfenfluramine but to learn from these experiences and not repeat mistakes. Prescribing a weight-loss medication for an individual patient will always be a unique decision. There are only two choices: prescribe or not prescribe. Each of these choices has ethical implications, and there is no way to escape the responsibility of making a decision. A decision to treat or not treat obesity with medication will ultimately reflect a physician's professional values and the patient's personal values.

■ Applicable Ethical Principles

The field of medical ethics does not offer a clear answer to the question of whether or not to prescribe, but it may provide a theoretical framework in which to think about the issue. The concepts of beneficence, nonmalfeasance, autonomy, informed consent, and professionalism are relevant to the decisions of when and how to prescribe weight loss medications.

Beneficence

Some physicians hold the principle of **beneficence**, doing what is best for the patient as the primary guiding principle of their practice. The clinician thus has an ethical obligation to consider a therapy if he or she has reason to believe that it will "help" the patient. The clinician must try to answer the question: will weight loss medications be of benefit to this particular person? The clinician should neither overestimate nor underestimate the potential benefits of the medications for that person.

Nonmalfeasance

The "flip side" of this issue is the principle of **nonmalfeasance**, the Hippocratic ethic to "first do no harm." Here the clinician must ask him- or herself what are the real risks of the therapy. Again the clinician should neither overestimate nor underestimate the risks. The role of the healthcare provider in this value system is to weigh these risks and benefits of therapy and make a judgment for the patient on the best course of action, using his or her expert judgment, professional experience, and the best information available.

■ Risks and Benefits

Before prescribing a weight-loss medication consider:

1. What degree of weight loss will likely be produced by the medication
2. What are the likely benefits of this weight loss for this person?
3. What are the risks of the medication for this patient?

Many of these issues are discussed in detail in chapter 14, but we do not have definitive answers for most of these questions. While the weight loss with existing medications is generally in the range of 5 to 10% of baseline weight, some individual lose more and others lose less. It is clear that markers of metabolic diseases—such as LDL cholesterol, insulin, and glucose levels, and, in some, blood pressure—are improved when overweight individuals are treated with these medications. Long-term risks appear to be minimal, and both sibutramine (Meridia) and orlistat (Xenical) have been used for many years in a large number of patients. While phentermine has been available for more than 30 years, and has been used in a large number of individuals world-wide, there have to date been no long-term safety or efficacy trials with this medication. In the European Union there is increasing pressure to remove phentermine from the market because of the availability of newer medications that have had more extensive testing, but the higher cost of the newer medications may price them out of reach for many poorer patients.

In deciding whom to treat with weight-loss medications, several factors should be considered. The first is that the health risks of obesity increase as the BMI increases. This means that the use of weight-reducing medications is probably not warranted purely for "health benefits" below a certain level of obesity. The FDA has set this level at a BMI of 30 for those without health complications and 27 for those with health complications. The second issue is that the absolute health risks of obesity rise as the individual ages. A 30-year-old woman with a BMI of 36 has an increased risk of dying of coronary artery disease, but this event is not likely to happen in the next 5 to 10 years. On the other hand, a 48-year-old individual with the same BMI is in more danger over the next 3 to 5 years. This means that the absolute benefit of medications probably is greater in older individuals. The third issue is that, in order to be beneficial, drug treatment of obesity will likely need to be long term. If the risk of side effects is higher with longer exposure, then the risk-benefit ratio would be more favorable in older individuals. Health risks of obesity are greater if the individual has a family history of health conditions associated with obesity, like hypertension, diabetes, and coronary artery disease. These factors suggest that the risk-benefit ratio associated with prescribing medications for weight loss is less in those with BMI less than 30 and younger than 30 years of age. As a person ages, becomes heavier, and either develops associated medical problems or has a family history of medical problems, the risk-benefit ratio moves in a direction that would favor treatment. Where an individual clinician will draw the line will be based on clinical judgment, but each clinician needs to draw a line somewhere.

■ Non-health Benefits of Weight Loss

Many patients who ask for weight-loss medications see their weight not as a health issue but as a quality-of-life issue. Other individuals are troubled by constant cravings for food and hope that an anorectic medication may help with these obsessive thoughts. What about these non-health benefits of weight-loss medications? Should these be given some weight in the risk-benefit calculation? This is a very difficult issue. While there is no doubt that using medications for these non-health benefits allows people to feel that they are doing something for their health, it is important not to promise weight loss that the patient will not experience or sustain. Many patients have unrealistic expectations about the amount of weight they will lose, and the degree to which that weight loss will improve their life. There is a fine line to negotiate between maintaining a realistic sense of hope and control on the part of the patient and providing honest expectations of the weight loss medications. Dealing realistically with patient expectations and goals (outlined in chapter 5) goes a long way toward providing truly informed consent. In a number of clinical trials using weight-loss medications, the drop-out rates at 1 and 2 years have been substantial. It is not known why the subjects dropped out, but it is possible that the weight loss provided proved less than many of these subjects had expected. While it is reasonable to consider non-health benefits of weight loss medications in a risk-benefit calculation, may ultimately lead to disappointment for both patient and provider.

On the other hand, most clinicians are comfortable prescribing Viagra for impotence or a serotonin-specific re-uptake inhibitor for patients in an effort to improve their quality of life. Physicians do not require documentation of "health benefits" before prescribing these medications. Patients often tell their doctor that they think a weight-loss medication will make it easier for them to stick to their diet. Their doctors may say, "Stick to your diet, then we can talk about medications." Physicians do not routinely withhold anti-diabetic medications just because a patient is not adhering to dietary recommendations. Why do the same physicians require rigid adherence to a behavioral program before considering weight loss medications? Are weight-loss medications being held to a different standard in this situation? If so, why?

■ Patient Autonomy

While the physician plays a role in weighing risks and benefits, the patient too plays an important role in this decision. The ethical principle of **autonomy** holds that the patient is a fully competent and independent person with a right to make decisions relevant to his or her health. One interpretation of this principle is that the patient should be the sole decision-maker in the doctor-patient relationship. Autonomy is a core professional value that guides many health care providers in the care they deliver. In this construction, that the healthcare provider has a responsibility to provide information and insure the decision made by the patient is an informed one, but the values and goals of the healthcare provider should not be substituted for those of the patient. The importance of patient autonomy is made clear in the context of difficult "end-of-life" decisions, where it is easier to see the importance of allowing a patient to refuse care. However, just as the principles of beneficence and non-malfeasance can be carried to an extreme, the principle of patient autonomy is carried to an extreme when the rights and responsibilities of the prescribing physician are overlooked. Problems caused by a focus solely on patients' rights were highlighted during the period when fen/phen (the commonly prescribed combination of phentermine and fenfluramine) was popular. During this period, many patients forcefully requested medications that clinicians were uncomfortable prescribing. Some clinicians chose to say no to patient demands, believing that risks outweighed benefits. However, given that autonomy was a strong guiding principle, many took the course of attempting to inform patients of risks and benefits, allowing the patient to decide whether or not to take the medications. While this general approach was uncomfortable for many, it reflected a fundamental commitment to patient autonomy. When it turned out that there were serious side effects to these medications, many clinicians felt patients were allowed to put too much pressure and pay too little regard to clinician judgment.

Perhaps the principle of autonomy means more than patient control of decision-making. An alternative view is that, in a doctor-patient relationship, autonomy implies that *both* the patient and the health care provider have "veto power," and embarking on any treatment requires that both the patient and the physician agree that the treatment is indicated, and both agree that risks outweigh benefits. A physician has no obligation to provide therapy that does not have a favorable risk-benefit ratio; in fact, there exists professional obligation to discourage a patient from embarking on such a course. Conversely, if a treatment is indicated, a physician must provide therapy knowing that even if a complication occurs, the best judgement of both parties was used in reaching that decision. Physician and patient have a joint responsibility to make independent risk/benefit assessments regarding the use of the weight loss medication.

■ Informed Consent

At the very core of the ethical responsibility to discuss risks and benefits is the process of **informed consent**. Each physician provides informed consent for diagnostic procedures and medications every day. For most interventions the process of informed consent is relatively informal. During the period when fen-phen was being prescribed, however, many healthcare providers struggled with how to more formally provide informed consent. Many developed and required patients to sign informed consent documents before receiving medication. Some of these documents were designed primarily to protect the physician from litigation. The focus of these documents was not an in-depth discussion of what was known about the effectiveness versus the health risks of these medications, but rather the patient was asked to relinquish any right to hold the practitioner responsible for adverse outcomes. A second kind of consent form appeared to be designed to scare patients out of decisions to use these medicines. These documents tended to minimize any potential benefits of the medications and exaggerate the risks. Neither of these types of documents fulfill the ethical responsibility to provide informed consent. An informed consent document cannot remove the culpability of the healthcare provider, who has a "fiduciary responsibility to patients to act in utmost good faith and to exercise due care." Healthcare workers cannot ethically or morally escape the professional responsibility of providing advice to patients. If a patient experiences a bad outcome as a result of a prescription that is written, there is some culpability. If a potentially beneficial medication is withheld because of a misrepresentation of risk, there is also culpability. An informed consent document should provide accurate and reliable information on risks and benefits to patients; no more, no less. It may be that an informed consent form is still the best approach that a busy primary care provider can use to fulfill the ethical responsibility to completely inform patients. Information sheets which clearly and neutrally outline risks and benefits but do not require a signature prior to actual prescribing may be a reasonable alternative approach.

■ Professionalism

How might issues of professionalism impact on the decision to prescribe weight-loss medications? Professionalism in the field of medicine has long been interpreted as putting the interest of the patient before the self-interest of the care provider. Much of the decline in the public image of the field of medicine can be traced to a public perception that physicians have placed personal financial gain over the best interests of patients. No one understands the primary motivating force better than the physician providing the service. Any physician who provides pharmacologic treatment for overweight or obese patients with a primary goal of gaining personal wealth is behaving in an unprofessional manner. Very few physicians knowingly do this, but their impact can be large.

More common is the physician who provides services that he or she believes are medically indicated but adopts practice habits that create the perception of a practice primarily driven by profit. Some weight-loss clinics which focus on treating obese or overweight patients may use certain practices which, while they do not constitute unprofessional behaviors, do raise questions in the minds of others about the motives of the practitioner. These include dispensing medications out of the practice for a fee and for profit, seeing a daily volume of patients that implies minimal physician contact with each patient, using medications for indications that are far from the mainstream (such as thyroid hormone in those with normal thyroid function tests, and diuretics purely for weight loss), and treating patients that other clinics might not, such as very young individuals or those with BMIs less then 25. A consistent pattern of these practice behaviors does raise questions as to the motive of practitioner.

■ Off-label Prescriptions

Contrary to what many patients think, the benefits of weight-loss medications appear to last only as long as the medications are taken. However, current labeling only allows for the use of phentermine and other older anorectic medications for three months. Sibutramine (Merida) currently has FDA approval for one year, although two-year safety and effectiveness data have been generated. Use beyond this time frame is not clearly sanctioned by the FDA. These FDA labeling issues create ethical problems in prescribing phentermine for longer than three months or sibutramine for greater than one or two years. Long-term prescriptions of these drugs might be considered "off-label" prescriptions. The use of medications for non-FDA approved indications has historically led to improved care in a number of medical conditions. For example, the use of beta blockers for angina and methotrexate for rheumatoid arthritis were initially off-label. Off-label prescriptions are commonplace and at times have been considered innovative therapies to reflect the fact that they are being given with the primary goal of improving patient health and that a drug may have therapeutic potential without FDA approval. Still, off-label prescriptions can generate a negative perception in the mind of care providers, and physicians using medications this way should be aware that there may be some legal culpability in the event of an adverse outcome. Prescribing a medication in a manner not specifically approved by the FDA is legal as long as the rationale for prescribing is clearly thought out and clearly explained to the patient, and that these steps are clearly documented in the medical record.

■ Reaching a Decision

Some physicians decide never to prescribe weight loss medications. Others prescribe them at the will of the patient. These are the ends of the spectrum. There is no one correct approach. Each physician should strive to engage these issues in the spirit of professionalism that Edmund Pelligrino of the Center for Clinical Bioethics at Georgetown University Medical Center describes as "the suppression of self-interest to that of the patient." When in doubt, discuss the issue with respected colleagues. If peers disagree with the approach you are taking, then you might discuss your reasoning with these individuals to more clearly understand the nature of the disagreement. Ultimately each physician has the moral authority and responsibility to decide how to care for patients. These decisions are not necessarily clear or easy. However, the lessons learned from a careful consideration of the ethical issues involved in the prescription of weight loss medications apply to many of the prescriptions that are written for other conditions every day in the office, prescriptions that are too often written without any consideration.

References

1. Pellegrino ED: Patient and physician autonomy: conflicting rights and obligations in the physician-patient relationship. J Contemp Health Law Policy 10:47-68, 1994.
2. Wynia MK, Latham SR, Kao AC, Berg JW, Emanuel LL: Medical professionalism in society. NEJM 341:1612-1616, 1999.
3. Ethics manual, 4th ed: American College of Physicians. Ann Intern Med 128:569-571, 1998.
4. Shelton JD: A piece of my mind: the harm of "first do no harm." JAMA 284:2687-2688, 2000.

Chapter 16

Robert Kushner, MD

Surgical Treatment of Obesity

Bariatric surgery should be considered for patients with severe obesity (BMI >40 kg/m^2) or those with moderate obesity (BMI >35 kg/m^2) associated with a serious medical problem. A 1991 NIH Consensus Development Conference Panel recognized two operative approaches—vertical banded gastroplasty (VBG) and Roux-en-Y gastric bypass (RYGB) (see figures). By limiting the storage capacity of the stomach to 30 to 50 cm and reducing the pouch-emptying rate by creation of a 10-mm diameter anastamotic gastrointestinal stoma, these two gastric restrictive surgeries significantly reduce the total volume and rate at which food can be consumed. The RYGB further limits caloric intake by inducing a "dumping syndrome" whenever sugar is consumed. These procedures are generally effective in producing an average weight loss of approximately 50% of excess body weight that is maintained in nearly 60% of patients at 5 years. Due to the complexity and chronicity of morbid obesity, all patients should be evaluated by a multidisciplinary team that incorporates medical, nutritional, and psychological care. The medical management of the bariatric surgical patient is a continual process, beginning with a thorough preoperative evaluation and continuing into the postoperative period to ensure long-term success.

Preoperative evaluation includes assessing and treating medical complications of obesity and assessing of the patient's ability to understand and comply with the postoperative regimen. The most common reasons for surgical exclusion are mental health disorders, including severe depression, schizophrenia, personality disorder, and substance abuse. For this reason a formal psychiatric evaluation is a standard part of the preoperative testing at many centers. Patients should receive dietary instruction before the operation in order to prepare their home with the foods and kitchen appliances—e.g., blender and measuring cups—needed immediately upon discharge from the hospital. Management of the patient during the immediate postoperative period is primarily directed toward reducing the risk for atelectasis, pneumonia, thromboembolic disease, and wound infections. In our program, patients are prescribed clear liquids on postoperative day 1 and advanced to a pureed diet on day 3 or 4 prior to hospital discharge.

Short-term (first six months) and long-term medical management of the bariatric patient encompasses treatment of ongoing chronic medical problems, monitoring for operative complications, and managing the known nutritional deficiencies that stem from the surgical procedures. Significant and rapid improvement in diabetes control, sleep apnea, hypertension, gas-

FIGURE 1. Vertical-banded gastroplasty

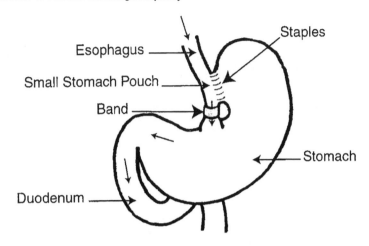

troesophageal reflux disease, urinary incontinence, and osteoarthritis, among others, are typically seen and may require tapering or discontinuation of medications. The most common surgical complications include stomal stenosis or marginal ulcers (occurring in 5%–15% of patients) that present as prolonged nausea and vomiting after eating or inability to advance the diet to solid foods. These complications are typically treated by endoscopic balloon dilatation and acid suppression therapy, respectively. Abdominal and incisional hernias (occurring in approximately 30% of patients) necessitate an operative repair, the timing of which is determined by symptoms and stabilization of body weight.

The nutritional implications of the VBG and RYGB procedures are predictable and should be treated proactively. Immediately after surgery, caloric intake is reduced to <1000 kcal/d, divided into multiple and small meals and snacks. Liquid and soft foods are prescribed for the first month and advanced to more solid foods thereafter. Beverages should be consumed apart from solid foods to allow greater intake of protein calories. For the first 6 months, patient nutritional counseling is focused on consumption of at least 60 grams of protein/day, primarily from dairy, egg, fish, poultry and soy, and ample use of dietary protein-fortified supplements. Over the first year, total caloric intake increases proportional to changes in pouch volume, stoma size, pouch-emptying rate, and increased consumption of solid food. Due to maldigestion, meat and dairy (in lactase-deficient patients) often remain poorly tolerated.

In general, mean weight loss is greater after the RYGB operation than after the VBG. This is thought to be due, in part, to development of the dumping syndrome. This syndrome represents a constellation of vasomotor and neuroendocrine events that collectively serve as negative reinforcers to

FIGURE 2. Roux-en-Y gastric bypass (RYGB)

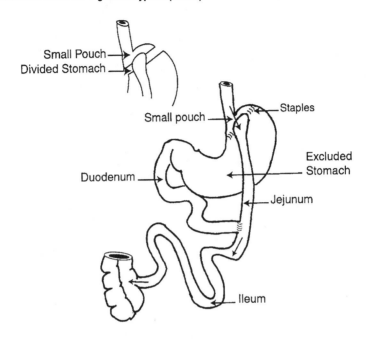

the consumption of simple sugars. The syndrome, which is initiated by rapid emptying of food into the jejunum, results in a variety of unpleasant and distressing symptoms including nausea, abdominal cramping, diarrhea, lightheadedness, tachycardia, flushing, and syncope. Although the symptom-induced intolerance to sugar-containing foods is a powerful incentive after surgery, the dumping syndrome often disappears within 12 to 18 months in many patients.

For patients who undergo a VBG, there are no intestinal absorptive abnormalities, other than mechanical reduction in gastric size and outflow. Therefore, selective deficiencies occur uncommonly unless eating habits remain restrictive and unbalanced. In contrast, the RYGB procedure produces a predictable increased risk for micronutrient deficiencies of vitamin B_{12}, iron, folate, and calcium based on surgical anatomic changes.

Cobalamin (vitamin B_{12}) deficiency has been reported to occur in >30% of patients 1 to 9 years after RYGB, since the procedure disrupts several of the key steps in vitamin B_{12} absorption. As a preventive measure, all patients should be orally supplemented with crystalline vitamin B_{12} in a daily dose of at least 350 g or receive monthly vitamin injections. Iron deficiency has been reported to occur in 33% to 50% of patients following RYGB and is more likely to occur in menstruating women. Folate deficiency occurs with a lower frequency than vitamin B_{12} or iron deficiency, but should be considered when evaluating a patient who develops anemia after RYGB. We typically prescribe one prenatal vitamin and mineral tablet daily for all of our RYGB patients to supply supplemental iron and folate. Iron deficient and anemic patients may require an additional iron supplement as well.

Calcium deficiency can result from several factors, including reduced intake of calcium- and vitamin D-containing foods, bypass of the duodenum, and malabsorption of vitamin D due to mismixing of pancreatic and biliary juices in the distal jejunum. For these reasons, RYGB patients may be at risk for developing osteoporosis or osteomalacia. In addition to periodic monitoring of serum calcium, phosphorus, alkaline phosphatase and 25(OH) vitamin D levels, all patients should receive calcium supplements of 1200 to 1500 mg/day in divided doses, depending on the adequacy of dietary calcium. Calcium citrate is the preferred preparation because it is more soluble than calcium carbonate in the absence of gastric acid production.

Bariatric surgery is now considered a well-established treatment for patients with clinically severe obesity. Patients can expect to lose approximately 1/3 of their initial body weight with resolution of co-morbid conditions and improvement in quality of life. Ongoing nutritional and medical management is required to prevent nutritional deficiencies and optimize post-operative care.

References

1. Kushner R: Managing the obese patient after bariatric surgery: a case report of severe malnutrition and review of the literature. Journal of Parenteral and Enteral Nutrition 24:126-132, 2000.
2. Balsiger BM, Luque-de Leon E, Sarr MG: Bariatric surgery for weight control in patients with morbid obesity. Med Clin North Am 84(2):477-489, 2000.
3. NIH Consensus Development Conference Panel: gastrointestinal surgery for severe obesity. Ann Intern Med 115:956-961, 1991.

Chapter 17

Holly R. Wyatt, MD, Rena R. Wing, PhD, and James O. Hill, PhD

The National Weight Control Registry

Just about everyone now recognizes that an epidemic of obesity exists in the United States and that obesity is a serious threat to health and quality of life. Despite this recognition there is still an overwhelming pessimism among health care professionals about the successful long-term management of obesity. Clinicians recognize the seriousness of obesity and know that weight loss would benefit their obese patients, yet most believe that ultimately their patients will fail at losing weight.

Is failure in weight management inevitable? In truth, the prevalence of long-term weight loss success in the general population of Americans needing to lose weight may not be nearly as "hopeless" as previously reported to the medical community. In a recent random-digit, telephone-based survey of 500 US adults, over 38% of subjects who had been overweight or obese reported that they were currently 10% below their maximum lifetime weight. NIH clinical guidelines specify that achieving a 10% reduction in body weight for obese patients will significantly improve health.

More optimism about success in long-term weight management can be seen in results from The National Weight Control Registry (NWCR). The NWCR was founded in 1994 by Drs. Rena Wing and James Hill with the idea that some people do succeed at long-term weight loss and that we could learn from their successes. The NWCR consists of over 3000 subjects who have maintained a minimum weight loss of 30 lbs. for at least one year, many for much longer. These successful "losers" are "winners" by any standard.

The purpose of this chapter is to summarize some of the behaviors that NWCR subjects have in common and to consider how this information may be useful in helping more overweight and obese patients to be successful in long-term weight maintenance.

■ Participants in the National Weight Control Registry

Currently over 3000 subjects in the NWCR are being followed for successful weight loss. The majority (80%) of NWCR participants are women, 97% are Caucasian, and 67% are married. The average registry member is 45 years of age and reports losing 67 lbs. and keeping at least 30 lbs. off for 5.5 years. Many (16%) have maintained at least a 30 lb. weight loss for greater than 10 years.

NWCR members also report a lifetime history of obesity. Forty-six percent of NWCR subjects report being overweight before the age of 12 years old and 72% report being overweight before the age of 18 years old. In addition, the majority of NWCR subjects (90%) have experienced unsuccessful past attempts at weight loss. Many also report a strong family history for obesity, with 46% reporting having one overweight or obese parent and 27% reporting both parents being overweight or obese.

■ Weight Loss vs. Weight Maintenance

One important finding is that there is more consistency in maintaining weight loss over time than in the method of initial weight loss. It is important to note that 89% of these subjects used both diet and exercise to achieve weight loss. Only 10% of these successful individuals lost weight by diet alone. This contrasts the commercial weight management area where diet seems to be given much more emphasis than physical activity. There was no consistent diet used for weight loss among successful NWCR individuals. Some used very low calorie diets, some counted calories, some counted fat, and some restricted certain foods. No particular type of diet was associated with more success in weight loss than any other.

About half of the NWCR subjects used a formal weight loss program (e.g., Weight Watchers) and about half lost weight on their own. Interestingly, the majority of men (63%) lost weight on their own while the majority of women (60%) used a formal program. Whether or not a formal program was used did not affect long-term success in weight maintenance.

■ Behaviors Common to Successful "Losers"

We found much more similarity in how NWCR subjects are maintaining a weight loss. We have identified four behaviors that are common to a large number of NWCR subjects.

1. NWCR subjects report eating a low-fat, high-carbohydrate diet. This is interesting given the current popularity of the low-carbohydrate and high-protein diets. In fact, <1% of NWCR subjects report eating a diet consistent with the popular Atkins' diet. On average, NWCR subject report eating a diet that is 24% fat, 19% protein, and 56% carbohydrate. The majority of meals were eaten at home, but these individuals were able to maintain weight loss while still occasionally enjoying meals eaten out.

2. NWCR subjects regularly monitor their weight and their food intake. About 75% of NWCR members weigh themselves weekly and 44% weigh themselves daily. Half of the registry members report that they keep track of energy (or fat) eaten on a regular basis. Thus, self-monitoring appears to be an important ongoing strategy for many of these successful losers.

3. NWCR subjects eat breakfast almost every day. 78% of registry members report that they eat breakfast every day. Only 4% report that they never eat breakfast.

4. NWCR subjects regularly engage in high levels of physical activity. Engaging in high levels of physical activity is a behavior seen in most NWCR subjects. On average, women in the registry report that they currently engage in 2545 kcal/week of physical activity and men engage in an average of 3293 kcal/week in physical activity. This amount of physical activity is comparable to walking 28 miles/week or about an hour per day of moderate-intensity physical activity. This amount of physical activity is much higher than physical activity recommendations for the general public. The Surgeon General recommends that adults engage in 30 minutes/day of moderate intensity physical activity on most day but at least 3 days/week.

Figure 1 shows the types of physical activity reported by NWCR members. Twenty-eight percent reported using only walking as their physical activity. Almost half report that they walk and engage in some additional form of physical activity. Fourteen percent report using only another form of regular exercise and not walking. Interestingly, only 9% report no regular physical activity.

Since most subjects report getting a large amount of their physical activity by walking, the activity level of NWCR members was also reported as steps/day by wearing a pedometer. On average, NWCR had over 11,000 steps/day. For comparison, a group of obese individuals were also evaluated by pedometer prior to starting a weight loss program. This group averaged only 5000 steps/day. These results suggest that subjects in the NWCR are engaging in substantially more stepping activities (such as walking or running) than obese subjects prior to weight loss.

Subjects in the NWCR report engaging in a large variety of activities. Table 1 shows the six most frequently reported physical activities of subjects in the registry. Walking was the most popular single activity. Seventy-seven

FIGURE 1. Classification of NWCR Members into Physical Activity Categories

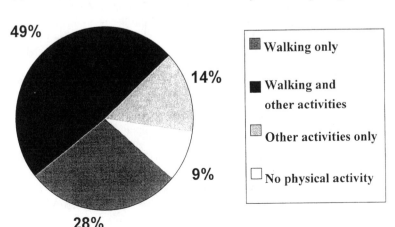

Table 1. The Six Most Frequently Reported Activities for NWCR Members

Activity	Males	Females	All
Walking	78.6%	76.1%	76.6%
Cycling	22.4%	20.2%	20.6%
Weight Lifting	24.0%	19.5%	20.3%
Aerobics	4.1%	20.9%	17.8%
Running	27.6%	14.2%	16.8%
Stair Climbing	3.1%	9.5%	9.3%

percent of registry members reported walking daily. One thing that stands out is the high proportion of NWCR women who engage in weight lifting. In the registry, 24% of men and 20% of women regularly engage in weight lifting. In the general population, 20% of men and only about 9% of women regularly engage in weight lifting. Thus women in the registry engaged in weight lifting to a much greater extent than women in the general population. It is not clear whether weight lifting contributes to the success of NWCR women, but this finding is being pursued to determine if it is advisable to recommend more resistance training for overweight and obese patients.

■ Can Physicians Use This Information for Patients?

First, all of the data obtained in the NWCR is correlational, and there is no certainty that the behaviors these subjects reported were factors in their success. However, the information obtained from these subjects is consistent with what is known about weight loss and weight loss maintenance. With this caveat, how can clinicians use this information?

Helping Patients Lose Weight

There is no identifiable optimum diet or diet strategy for weight loss. This is interesting, given the interest of the general public in finding exactly the right kind of diet that "really works." Perhaps the type of diet used is not as important as the fact that total calories are reduced and perhaps different people do better on different types of diets. Data show that only 10% of NWCR subjects achieved their weight loss by diet alone. This suggests that it might be a reasonable strategy for patients to modify both diet and physical activity to lose weight. Currently there seems to be more emphasis on diet than on physical activity in weight management.

Helping Patients Maintain a Weight Loss

Should clinicians be telling obese patients to eat low fat, high carbohydrate diets, frequently monitor their weight and food intake, eat breakfast every day, and engage in an hour each day of physical activity? We cannot say with certainty that these behaviors were the cause of the success seen in these NWCR members. Indeed, some people were maintaining a weight loss without engaging in any regular physical activity. There seems to be no single formula for success in weight loss maintenance, and yet there was surprising consistency in the types of behaviors used. Only 1% were eating a low carbohydrate diet, only 25% did not weigh themselves at least weekly, only 4% did not eat breakfast, and only 9% were not exercising regularly. These behaviors are consistent with the few other studies of long-term weight loss success, so it can at least be concluded that the odds favor those who engage in these behaviors.

A low-fat diet may be more important in weight maintenance than in weight loss. Several studies have shown that total energy intake is lower when subjects are allowed to self-select food intake from low-fat as opposed to high-fat foods, yet lowering the fat content of the diet is associated with only a small amount of weight loss (usually 1-2 kg). Thus, while eating a low-fat diet may not produce large amounts of weight loss, it does seem to be associated with a slightly lower food intake and may be helpful in avoiding weight gain.

Self-monitoring of body weight and food intake is a factor that has been identified by others as being associated with successful weight loss maintenance. Frequent weighing may be associated with early detection of weight gain, allowing the subject to take corrective action to prevent further weight gain. Frequent monitoring of food intake may serve to focus attention on food choices and prevent overeating.

There is less information available about breakfast eating and long-term success in weight-loss maintenance. Many formal weight loss programs focus on eating breakfast as a way of reducing hunger later in the day.

Finally, physical activity is consistently associated with long-term success in maintaining a reduced body weight. Most subjects (91%) in the NWCR report engaging in regular physical activity to maintain their weight loss. Most NWCR subjects far exceed the Surgeon General's recommendation for 30 minutes of exercise most days of the week. Only 9% of registry subjects report that they are maintaining their weight loss without regular physical activity.

■ Is Life Better After Weight Loss?

Some experts have been concerned that weight loss and the vigilance required to maintain weight loss long-term may have negative psychological consequences. No adverse psychological effects of weight loss (eating disorders, depression, etc.) have been observed in the National Weight Control Registry. In fact, rates of binge eating and vomiting are strikingly lower than what is observed in populations with eating disorders. Further, over 90% of NWCR members report improvements in their overall quality of life, level of energy, mobility, general mood, self-confidence, and physical health after weight loss.

■ Summary

The perception that people rarely succeed at long-term weight loss is not true. Results from the National Weight Control Registry show that successful weight loss maintenance is possible. This does not mean that all patients will lose as much weight as these successful "losers." Maintaining weight loss is difficult and seems to be a lifelong challenge. This chapter provided some suggestions for how to help patients be more successful in long-term weight loss maintenance. These are not sure formulas for success but they can help achieve long-term weight loss maintenance, and patients really need help in achieving these behaviors. In today's world it is difficult to eat a low fat diet and engage in physical activity for an hour each day. The challenge may not be as much in knowledge of what to do as in execution. Clinicians can be helpful in identifying behaviors associated with long-term weight maintenance success, but most patients will need considerable help in making permanent behavior changes.

Additional Reading

1. Kayman S, Bruvold W, Stern, JS: Maintenance and relapse after weight loss in women: behavioral aspects. Am J Clin Nutr 52:800-807, 1990.
2. Klem ML, Wing RR, McGuire MT, Seagle HM, Hill JO: A descriptive study of individuals successful at long-term maintenance of substantial weight loss. Am J Clin Nutr 66:239-246, 1997.
3. Schoeller DA, Shay K, Kushner RF:. How much physical activity is needed to minimize weight gain in previously obese women? Am J Clin Nutr 66:551-6, 1997.
4. Wing RR, Hill JO: Successful weight loss maintenance. Annu Rev Nutr 21:323-41, 2001.

Chapter 18

Thomas N. Robinson, MD, MPH

Primary Care Management of Pediatric Obesity

It is easy to list reasons *not* to manage overweight children in primary care settings. Insufficient time and assessment/counseling skills may cause the provider to question his or her effectiveness in this arena. Inadequate reimbursements from third-party payers and a lack of organizational or health system support (e.g., staff support and resources) can frustrate even the most committed provider. Providers also may be deterred by uncertainty about the efficacy of the interventions they have to offer—from their past frustrations treating overweight patients or from trying to control their own weight. Finally, a lack of both provider and patient knowledge or insight into the magnitude of the problem may allow it to remain an unaddressed facet of primary care.

Still, there are equally or more compelling reasons *to* manage overweight children in primary care settings.

1. Rates of obesity are rising at epidemic rates among children in the U.S. and throughout the world. As a result, primary care providers are seeing more and more overweight children. Although they do not always intervene, some primary care providers now estimate obesity to be the most common problem they see in their practices.

2. Recent data suggest that many overweight children manifest substantial obesity-related morbidities that are not detected. Among 5 to 17-year-old children participating in the Bogalusa Heart Study in Bogalusa, Louisiana, about 60% of overweight children already had at least one additional cardiovascular disease risk factor: hypertension, elevated total cholesterol, elevated low-density lipoprotein cholesterol, low high-density lipoprotein cholesterol, elevated triglycerides, or elevated insulin level.

3. Pediatric primary care providers are credible sources of health-related information and advice for their patients.

4. Pediatric providers are already familiar with normal childhood and adolescent behavior and development, allowing them to incorporate developmentally appropriate behavioral messages and strategies more easily than other health professionals.

5. Primary care providers have greater exposure to children than other health professionals in the form of both periodic health maintenance examinations and acute illness visits. These visits provide the opportunity to evaluate and manage weight problems earlier rather than later.

6. Parents or guardians are already present at children's primary care visits, allowing evaluation and interventions to involve the parents or guardians in addition to the children. Pediatric primary care providers are also accustomed to addressing behavioral problems within the social and family context.

7. There is reason to be optimistic about the potential efficacy of primary care interventions for weight control. While data are scarce for weight control interventions per se, there are data suggesting some short-term efficacy of primary care–based interventions for other health behaviors, such as smoking cessation.

Once primary care providers decide to substantively address the issue of pediatric obesity, they need an effective and efficient way to do so. Unfortunately, the evidence base is limited regarding practical approaches to evaluation and treatment of overweight children. Recommendations based on the existing literature and on the experience of a number of experienced researchers and clinicians, however, are available.[1] These "expert committee" recommendations, in addition to reviews of the most effective behavioral treatment strategies[2] and the author's personal experiences as a general pediatrician, form the basis of the practical strategies suggested below.

■ Evaluation of the Overweight Child

Identification and Measurement

The first step in evaluation of the overweight child is identification of significant overweight. The body mass index (BMI) is considered the best screening method for detecting overweight among children and adolescents.[3] BMI is calculated as the weight (measured in kilograms) divided by the square of the height (measured in meters) as shown in Table 1.

BMI tables and calculators are widely available in printed form and for computers, palm computers, and on the internet. BMI requires only the accurate measurement of height and weight, and is correlated with more direct measures of body fatness and clinical morbidity. Occasionally an elevated BMI may be due to an extraordinary amount of muscle, and not reflect increased fatness. In these cases, a measure of triceps skinfold thickness will help discriminate between overweight and overfat. The accurate measure of skinfold thickness, however, requires training and experience, and it is therefore not recommended for routine use in primary care settings. In almost all cases seen in primary care practices, overweight and overfat are synonymous. Other, more involved and

---

TABLE 1. Calculating Body Mass Index (BMI)

BMI = Weight in kilograms ÷ Height in meters ÷ Height in meters
      OR
BMI = (Weight in kilograms ÷ Height in centimeters ÷ Height in centimeters) × 10,000
      OR
BMI = (Weight in pounds ÷ Height in inches ÷ Height in inches) × 703

more expensive measures of body composition are not recommended, as they rarely add any additional useful information for the primary care provider.

Reference standards for BMI for age and sex are now available in the revised 2000 growth charts developed by the Centers for Disease Control and Prevention (CDC) (http://www.cdc.gov/growthcharts/). Children with a BMI at or above the reference 95th percentile for their age and sex are considered overweight, and recommended for evaluation and intervention. Children with a BMI at or above the reference 85th percentile but below the 95th percentile for their age and sex are considered at risk of overweight, and recommended for evaluation with possible intervention. These percentile thresholds roughly match the thresholds for obesity (BMI ≥ 30) and overweight (BMI ≥ 25) in adults, respectively.[3]

History and Physical Examination

All children who are overweight (≥ 95th percentile) or at risk of overweight (≥ 85th percentile) should receive a complete medical history and physical exam. The goals of this evaluation are to identify the small minority of children who may be overweight secondary to one of the rare metabolic or genetic causes of obesity, to assess risks, and to identify complications of overweight or co-morbidities. A quick screen for rare causes of obesity includes short stature/poor growth in height, dysmorphic features, hypogonadism, and developmental delay or mental retardation. Overweight children with any of these four findings may be referred to a pediatric obesity specialty clinic or a pediatric endocrinologist or geneticist for further evaluation for metabolic and genetic causes. Overweight children without these four findings can be considered to be suffering from overnutrition, an excess of energy intake over energy expenditure. An insulin-secreting neoplasm can also cause obesity, but a child with this disorder would present with other signs and symptoms.

To help assess risks, the history and physical exam should include a review of growth patterns since early childhood, plotting the weight and height, the weight-for-height (prior to 2 years of age) and the BMI (after age 2 years), a family history of obesity, cardiovascular disease, hyperlipidemia, type 2 diabetes and obesity-associated complications, a social history, and a puberty history and a genital exam. A review of symptoms and physical exam should also include assessment of potential obesity-related complications and/or co-morbidities, of which there are many. Hypertension and type-2 diabetes are common. Acanthosis nigricans, a hyperpigmentation of the skin in the folds of the neck or the axillae, is often associated with hyperinsulinemia and insulin resistance. Obstructive sleep apnea or obesity hypoventilation syndrome may manifest as snoring and restless sleeping and/or daytime somnolence, and may be associated with enlarged tonsils and adenoids. Pseudotumor cerebri may present with headaches and/or blurred optic discs on a retinal exam. Cholelithiasis should be considered with colicky abdominal pain and tenderness. Polycystic ovary disease, may manifest with menstrual disorders and hirsutism. Slipped capital femoral epiphysis may appear as hip or knee pain and limited range of motion, and Blount's disease (tibia vara) is a bowing of the tibia. Finally, eating disorders, which may manifest as binge eating and/or purging, or other psychological and social morbidities, such as depression, a change in family structure, teasing by other children, or a history of abuse or neglect many become evident on further questioning. Most of these conditions will require referral to an appropriate specialist for further evaluation and management.

The only laboratory studies recommended for all overweight children are screening fasting serum glucose (to detect type-2 diabetes), and a lipoprotein panel (to detect dyslipidemias). A fasting insulin can be obtained to detect hyperinsulinemia but is not mandatory. Identification of any of these abnormalities may provide greater motivation for the patient and family to make behavioral changes. Additional studies are only recommended as guided by findings from the history and physical exam (e.g., sleep study to diagnose sleep apnea, ultrasound exam to diagnose cholelithiasis, radiographs to diagnose slipped capital femoral epiphysis or Blount's disease). Thyroid function tests are not indicated routinely, as hypothyroidism is highly unlikely in a child with normal growth in height and no other signs or symptoms. In the case of a family that refuses to accept that their child's overweight is not due to a "glandular" or metabolic cause, however, thyroid function tests may help provide some reassurance.

Deciding Whether or Not to Treat

It has been recommended that overweight children over the age of 2 years (BMI ≥ 95th percentile for age and sex) receive some form of treatment for either weight maintenance (2 to 7 year olds with no obesity-related complications) or weight loss (2 to 7 year olds with an obesity-related complication and overweight 7+ year olds with or without an obesity-related complication).[1] However, other factors may also be taken into account by the clinician to determine the timing and intensity of treatment. As with all medical treatments there are potential side effects even when treatment is supervised by a health professional. These include linear growth retardation from nutritional insufficiency, arrhythmias that have been associated with very-low-calorie diets, the possible adverse effects of weight cycling or yo-yo dieting, and of course the economic, professional, and emotional costs of the long-term treatment of a chronic disease like obesity. On the other hand, there are other factors that encourage more immediate and intensive treatment. These factors are listed in Table 2.

Children who are already manifesting medical, social, or psychological obesity-related complications or co-morbidities are in need of more timely treatment. Sleep apnea and obesity hypoventilation syndrome are potentially life-threatening complications of obesity, and require rapid weight loss and often other concurrent treatments. Children with hypertension, dyslipidemias, or hyperinsulinemia may also require more rapid weight loss to improve those risk factors.

TABLE 2. Factors Encouraging Treatment

Presence of medical complications and/or co-morbidities

Presence of social or psychological complications and/or co-morbidities

Factors associated with greater risk of adult obesity
> greater BMI
> adolescent age group
> longer duration of overweight
> other overweight family members
> early adiposity rebound

Family history of cardiovascular diseases, type 2 diabetes, or other obesity-related morbidities

Abdominal fat distribution

Both child and parent(s) motivated

Other factors encouraging treatment are associated with a greater risk of future adult obesity. These include a greater BMI (the more overweight the greater the risk), older age (overweight adolescents are much less likely to grow into normal weight adults than overweight pre-pubertal children), a longer duration of overweight (a child who has been overweight for a longer period of years is less likely to become a normal weight adult), and the presence of other family members who are overweight. In addition, by charting BMI, primary care providers may be able to document what has been termed an early "adiposity rebound."[4] BMI growth charts reveal that the population BMI hits its low point between the ages of about 5 and 7 years of age. It has been shown that children who hit their BMI nadir early (before the age of about 5 or 5.5 years) and whose BMIs then start to climb are more likely to be overweight adults.

Overweight children who have a family history of heart disease, stroke, type-2 diabetes, or other obesity-related morbidities may also be at higher risk of those same complications as they grow older.

An abdominal predominance of body fat has been associated with greater risk of cardiovascular morbidity and mortality in adults. The data are less clear among children, complicated somewhat by the lack of easy, reliable, and valid measures. However, there may be some theoretical benefit to being more aggressive with treatment in a child with a distribution of body fat that favors the abdomen.

Finally, one of the most important factors to consider in deciding whether or not to start treatment and how intensely to pursue weight control is the level of child and parent motivation for weight control and behavior change. If either the child or parent is not ready to make a commitment to change behavior, treatment is much less likely to succeed, and the process will be much more frustrating for all persons involved (including the clinician). No one can deny that making significant lasting changes in behavior is difficult. In some cases, it may be better to delay treatment until a child and parent are ready to make changes or to help them become ready, rather than to push forward in an effort that is likely to fail.

■ Treating the Overweight Child

General Principles

Several general principles can be recommended for primary care treatment of obesity. First, **the child and parent must be ready to make changes in behavior**. In some cases, particularly for younger children, intervening with parents alone may be effective. In these cases, emphasis is put on things that parents have control over—the food environment of the home (e.g., what foods are available in the home), family eating behaviors (e.g., limiting eating out, serving portions from the kitchen instead of self-service at the dinner table), and parental responses to child behaviors (e.g., contingency management, as described below). These parent-instituted changes cannot be expected to help the child make more healthful choices at school or outside the home, where parents lack control over the environment. It is also important that parents avoid taking on the role of policing a child's eating and activity behaviors. This often leads to a new challenge for the child, to try to get around the limits set by the parent, that may prove more motivating to a child than just complying with the recommended behaviors. It is preferable to attempt treatment when both the child and the parent are both motivated to make changes. In cases where families are not motivated for treatment or there are conflicts between parent and child regarding food and or weight, referral for family therapy may be a useful prelude or adjunct to treatment.

A second general principle is that **childhood overweight is a chronic problem**, not something that can be "cured" with a quick fix. Once treatment is started, the clinician, parent, and child should expect it to continue for years. Most children become overweight over a span of years, and one may expect it to take as long or longer to achieve normal weight status. One way to illustrate the long-term nature of treatment to children and parents is with the child's weight growth chart. A horizontal line drawn to the right of the child's last measure illustrates how long it would take for the child to reach the median weight for age (or in some cases, just get back below the 95th percentile of weight for age) if they were to gain no additional weight. Even if a child is successful in controlling their weight in the short-term, maintaining a healthy weight is likely to be a lifelong challenge for them. As a result, **treatments should promote long-term, permanent behavior change**, and changes should be made slowly, in small incremental steps. Rapid, overnight changes rarely stick.

A third general principle is that **behavior change requires frequent feedback**. Feedback does not always have to be in the form of an office visit, but primary care providers should plan on scheduling frequent office visits or other opportunities to provide feedback. This is especially important during the early months of treatment, when new skills are being learned and new behavior change goals are being set. These early "visits" should be as frequent as weekly or every two weeks, if possible. To reduce some of the burden of such frequent visits, providers may also be able to take advantage of nurses, dietitians, social workers, psychologists, or health educators in their practice or their community, particularly if they are already trained in behavior change methods.

Behavioral Strategies

The core of primary care treatment of overweight children is helping families implement four behavioral strategies: controlling their environment, self-monitoring their behaviors, setting appropriate goals, and rewarding successful behavior change. **Controlling the environment** refers to reducing environmental cues and opportunities associated with increased calorie intake and inactivity, and increasing cues and opportunities for physical activity. These changes take two main forms: altering access and establishing new routines. Remove identified high-risk foods from the home and keep them out of the home. Reduce take-out meals or restaurant meals, where there is less control over what ingredients are used, how food is prepared, and the portions served. Prepare school lunches the night before instead of allowing children to buy their lunches from the *a la carte* service at school. Schedule time for routine family walks, bike rides, or recreational outings and establish a nightly meeting time to review the day's diet and activity behaviors and provide an opportunity to praise behavior change and problem solve around obstacles.

Self-monitoring is crucial to any behavior change effort. If a behavior cannot be measured reliably (i.e., counted) then it is difficult to set goals, judge whether or not there has been any change, provide feedback, or reward success. Therefore, behavior change efforts need to focus on behaviors that can be assessed or counted reliably. The typical general advice to reduce high fat foods and sweets and increase exercise is difficult to respond to, because most people cannot assess them reliably. In contrast, it is possible to count the number of fast food meals eaten, the number of soft drinks consumed, the number of desserts eaten, the number of days walked to school, or the number of vegetables consumed. Weight control treatments universally include self-monitoring and recording of targeted dietary behaviors and physical activity behaviors. There is evidence that self-monitoring alone produces some changes in behavior, and it is recommended that self-monitoring continue throughout the entire treatment period. After initial weight control it may become less frequent, although periodic self-monitoring is necessary to keep children and families on track, or get them back on track, during the maintenance phase of treatment as well.

Self-monitoring and **goal setting** go hand-in-hand. Appropriate goals can be set and monitored for success only if behaviors are being assessed reliably. Many children and their families want to lose lots of weight rapidly. However, to maintain adequate nutrition and growth and to promote long-term weight control, it is recommended that treatments focus on shorter-term behavior-change goals along with longer-term weight control goals. This makes appropriate goal setting crucial in pacing a family through changes in their behavior and maintaining their enthusiasm over a prolonged treatment period.

Rewarding successful behavior change is also tightly linked to self-monitoring and goal setting. This is also called contingency management, in which positive reinforcement is tied to specific behaviors. It is important for parents to learn that rewards should be frequent when children are first learning a new behavior, and then can become less frequent as the new behavior becomes established. It is also important that parents learn to be specific and consistent in their rewards and punishments. The same behavior should not be rewarded one time and discouraged another because mixed messages are counterproductive. Positive reinforcement also should be directed at the desired behavior, not at a general characteristic of the child. "I am very proud of you for going outside to play instead of sitting in front of the TV all afternoon," is more effective than "You are such a good child," which does not specify the behavior that prompted the praise. Parents often need guidance in choosing appropriate rewards as well. The magnitude of the reward should match the magnitude of the child's accomplishment. Praise and attention from a parent can be some of the most powerful and motivating rewards for children, and are usually more effective than material rewards. Parents should be encouraged to use their praise and attention as primary methods of rewarding their child's behavior. When children achieve their weekly behavioral goals, use rewards that involve activities that the children and parents perform together or extra privileges. Using food, expensive gifts (e.g., a new bicycle), or money is strongly discouraged. Contracts can also be used to help maintain focus on specific behavioral goals and to provide a structure for rewarding desired changes. Children and parents need to learn to negotiate realistic contracts (especially rewards they are willing and able to provide), to make contracts binding, not to alter the terms once a contract has been made (no renegotiations), and to provide agreed upon rewards as soon as possible after the goal has been achieved.

Assessing Diet and Activity

Essentially all weight control strategies involve approaches to reduce dietary energy intake and increase physical activity energy expenditure. An energy deficit may be produced by a number of different dietary changes, reducing total calories, such as reducing fat intake, increasing fiber intake, etc., or it can be attained with activity changes, such as increasing structured activities and/or lifestyle activities. Few data are available on the efficacy of different approaches. In the primary care setting, where time is limited, a brief dietary recall can serve to help guide the development of individual goals for dietary change. The purpose is *not* to fully characterize a child's diet, but to identify specific potential dietary targets for behavior change. A brief review of the current day's intake or a typical day's intake can serve to identify specific high-calorie foods (e.g., pizza every day at school, multiple pastries every morning, excessive amounts of soft drinks), high-calorie food preparation methods (e.g., frying in lard, butter, or margarine), a high prevalence of eating out and/or eating fast food (e.g., fast food for school lunches or dinners), or high-risk eating patterns (e.g., large snacks on the way home from school or after school, self-service at the dinner table) that may be susceptible to change.

Physical activity assessments similarly should be directed to identify specific potential activity targets for behavior change, not total calories expended. A brief assessment can review participation in organized sports classes, teams, or clubs, participation in physical education at school, methods of transportation to and from school, outdoor play after school and on weekends, and active chores. Sedentary behaviors should also be assessed. In particular, typical use of television, videotapes, DVDs, video games, computers, and talking on the phone, which may be targeted for decreases.

Short-term Diet and Activity Goals

Effective goals need to be simple and explicit, easy to measure, unambiguous, and not subject to interpretation. Therefore, explicit, easily counted behaviors are the best to target. Reduce by a specific number of times per day or week or eliminate specific foods that are identified in the diet screen. Change food preparation methods (by substituting grilling or minimum amounts of spray oils for frying) and reduce trips to fast food restaurants by a specific number of times per day or week. Set a goal to write down every time targeted foods are eaten. Representative physical activity examples include walking or biking to school a specific number of times per week, planning a family outdoor activity every Saturday and Sunday, walking a specific number of extra steps (using a pedometer) or blocks per day, or increasing by a specific number over the prior week. Definitely limit television, videotapes, and video games to one hour per day or seven hours per week.

Goals are usually more effective if they are chosen by the child instead of being imposed by the parent or clinician. The clinician and parent can help by proposing two or more choices and letting the child select the one they like the best—a behavior change they are willing to try and think they can achieve. Even if the goals originate from the clinician and/or parent, a child will be more motivated to achieve the goal if he or she perceives a choice in selecting that goal.

Finally, it is important to introduce new behavior-change goals gradually, only one or two at a time. The difficulty of the goal can be matched to the enthusiasm and confidence of the child and family, but it is important not to start with a goal that is too difficult. If too many goals are set too soon, a child and family can become overwhelmed, and are more likely to fail. Selected goals may be very small at first, such as reducing the number of fast food meals from 5 to 4 per week, or mixing milk as half whole milk and half 2% fat milk as the first step in moving from whole milk to non-fat milk. This is where the frequent visits and feedback become most important. Not only do families need help selecting appropriate behavior change goals but also in pacing their behavior change attempts to promote gradual but long-term changes.

Problem Solving

Once treatment is underway, a major role of the primary care provider is to help children and families problem solve, and to identify solutions to perceived barriers. Although solutions may seem obvious to others, families can find it difficult to find ways around barriers in their own family and lifestyle contexts. It could be that other family members or peers do not want to change, or there could be difficulty sticking with dietary goals when eating in others' homes, in restaurants, or attending birthday or holiday parties, and even intentional or unintentional sabotage from rival family members or loving grandmothers. Schools may offer few healthful choices for snacks or lunches. Children may experience hunger associated with boredom after school, and even eat as a coping response to stress. Parents may have safety concerns about allowing children to play outside. Potential barriers like these should be solved by families themselves, with the help of a clinician as needed. In the case of resistant family members or peers, and even saboteurs, families can identify motives to encourage the participation of other family members, and express to others the importance of weight control to the child. Children should be encouraged not to feel embarrassed about wanting to control their weight but, to the contrary, they should be praised for making such a responsible commitment to do something positive for themselves. If given the chance, the children themselves might come up with feasible and effective solutions to barriers. They could decide to ask their friends at school or their grandmothers to help them monitor and achieve their goals or to participate along with them. They often come up with many creative solutions to being faced with birthday cake or trick-or-treating, allowing them to participate but not consume all the cake and ice cream served or all the candy they collect (e.g., one piece per day for 10 days and throw away the rest, donate it all to a hospital or homeless shelter, etc.)

Teaching Parenting Skills

Too often, parents feel the need to police their child's eating and activity behaviors, trying to enforce dietary restrictions and activity goals. This usually backfires when children find it more challenging to avoid their parents' policing efforts than to comply with their goals (breaking the "rules" behind their backs, or even right to their face). To make lasting changes in behavior, children need to take responsibility themselves for making changes. A parent can help a child succeed by removing high-risk food from the home, offering low-calorie snacks, eating out less, altering food preparation methods, meeting nightly to review the day's diet and activity, and praising healthful behaviors, but it is not the parent's responsibility to make sure the child achieves his or her goals. Many parents find it very difficult, and even feel a sense of personal failure, if their child fails to achieve the goal. If the parent acts as if he or she is the one who is responsible for the child's eating and activity choices, the child never learns to make the changes. Some parents easily adapt to the supportive role while others need to be reminded over and over again that it is the child, not the parent, who has to take responsibility for eating less and being more active.

Other general parenting skills also should to be highlighted. First, parents need to be both consistent and contingent in their behavior toward their child. Some parents need to be taught to set limits, and how and when to say "no." Parents need to send consistent messages and their responses to their child's behaviors need to be contingent upon those behaviors. As noted above, praise, attention, rewards, and punishments should be tied to specific child behavior, and not applied inconsistently or without cause.

Second, parents need to be observant. If they are not aware of their child's behavior or if they are not paying attention, they cannot respond consistently and contingently.

Third, many parents need to be taught to use praise more effectively— specific to a behavior, not a general attribute of the child. It can even be helpful to ask parents to record the number of times and under what circumstances they praise their child each day to help set goals for improvement.

Fourth, teaching parents to use contracts effectively, as described above, can also be useful. Some weight loss programs teach children to make "reciprocal" contracts with their parents, to promote parent behavior changes that help them make their own changes. Parents set a goal (e.g., remove certain trouble foods from the house, go for a walk with their child every day after dinner, meet nightly, etc.) and parent and child negotiate a reward that the child will provide for the parent if the goal is achieved.

Fifth, parents need to be reminded that children learn much of their behavior by watching others, and parents themselves are the most important models in their child's life. "Do as I say, not as I do," does not work. As a result, parents need to model commitment to behavior change. Some parents also need to be encouraged to let their children see them fail every once in a while. Parents who never let their child see them fail never teach their children how to respond to adversity and to regroup and move forward. It is not uncommon to see a family with a long history of control issues and conflicts over food and eating. These conflicts often have to be addressed, or at least acknowledged and avoided, prior to making any progress on diet changes.

Finally, it is important to teach parents to meet frequently with their child. These meetings provide opportunities to review both child and parent behaviors, provide feedback (e.g., praise), set goals, negotiate contracts, monitor progress, discuss strategies to overcome barriers to change, and plan ahead.

Weight Goals

Short-term goals focus on diet and activity changes, while weight goals are often longer-term. There are differing opinions, and a paucity of data, on how aggressive to be in setting weight-loss goals. Therefore, an individual-ized approach to setting weight-loss goals is warranted. Children manifest-ing serious co-morbidities (e.g., slipped capital femoral epiphysis, severe obstructive sleep apnea) often require aggressive and immediate attempts to reduce weight (e.g., protein-modified fast, pharmacologic treatments, gastric bypass surgery) to minimize further morbidity and, in some cases, prevent mortality. Aggressive weight loss is best addressed by providers or centers that specialize in treating overweight children. A more gradual weight loss approach is recommended for the primary care setting, to promote longer-term success and prevent nutritional insufficiency and complications of weight loss.

Current recommendations suggest starting with a goal of weight mainte-nance. Coincident with normal growth in height, simply maintaining the same weight over time will result in reduced BMI. If actual weight loss is desired, an appropriate starting goal is about one pound weight loss per month. Again, coincident with normal growth in height, even a small reduc-tion in weight will substantially reduce BMI over time. At the primary care program at Stanford the goal is between no change in weight (weight main-tenance) and an average of one pound weight loss per week. This appears to be a realistic, safe, and motivating range for most children. If a child is con-sistently losing more than one pound per week the child's diet is reviewed to make sure the child is not overly restricting calories, skipping meals, or adopting other unhealthful behaviors. The long-term weight goal should be to achieve a BMI less than the 85th percentile for age and sex. Achievement of satisfactory weight loss can also be gauged along with improvements or resolution in accompanying co-morbidities, such as hyperlipidemia, hyper-insulinemia, acanthosis nigricans, hypertension, and hepatic steatosis.

Assessment of Treatment Progress and Potential Complications of Treatment

Progress should be monitored at every visit throughout the course of treat-ment. Review diet and activity records and progress towards achieving short-term behavior change goals. Revise goals if necessary and set new short-term behavior change goals. Measure (on the CDC growth charts), and provide feedback on changes in height, weight and BMI, and assess changes in any identified co-morbidities. Some children and families have trouble under-standing that because weight and BMI normally increase with age in chil-dren, even a slowed increase represents a reduction in overweight—progress they should feel proud of. To more clearly demonstrate improvements, one can also calculate and record changes in percent overweight (100 × [child BMI minus median BMI for age and sex] ÷ median BMI for age and sex). Seeing a reduction in percent overweight may be more motivating to a child and family than seeing a slowed increase or maintenance in BMI and weight.

Potential treatment complications should also be assessed at each visit. The most common side effects to look for are reduced growth in height, excessive weight loss, preoccupation with weight and body shape or adoption of unhealthy weight control behaviors (e.g., highly restrictive dieting, binge-eating, purging, use of diet pills, cathartics, or laxatives), and worsening parent-child or family functioning.

Reduction in height velocity is almost universally reported in response to weight control. This is somewhat expected because overweight children are usually tall for their age, so a modest reduction in height velocity is not thought to result in compromised adult height. However, severe growth retardation from nutritional insufficiency has been reported in children on restrictive diets. Gallbladder disease is another potential complication more likely to be seen in adolescents during rapid weight loss, and arrhythmias have been noted in association with weight loss using some very low calorie diets.

Disordered eating attitudes and behaviors are more common among overweight children, particularly among children and families seeking weight loss treatment. Therefore, it is important to assess for eating-disorders symptoms before starting treatment and throughout the course of treatment and follow-up.

Family behavior patterns are not always easily changed. Attempting and successfully changing child and parent behavior may result in dramatic changes in family interactions, leading to new problems in child-parent or family relationships. Therefore, some families may require referral for additional therapy to address these problems.

Long-term Maintenance of Weight Control

There has been little research to help guide successful long-term maintenance of weight control in children. As noted above, overweight should be treated as a chronic problem. Weight regain is very common, even after the most successful treatments. The same principles of behavior change still apply when addressing relapses. It is recommended that regular visits be continued. The optimal frequency is unknown, and may vary with the individual patient. Some children and families may require continued weekly or monthly visits to maintain their behavior changes and their weight loss, while others may require only twice-annual visits. To help address the need for continued contact, primary care providers may consider enlisting the participation of other health professionals to help them provide ongoing feedback and support to children and families. These could include dietitians, health educators, school nurses, social workers, public health nurses, etc. It will be important, however, that they share the same behavioral approaches so children and families receive a consistent message.

In addition to monitoring progress, reviewing behaviors and goals, setting new goals if needed, and assessing for potential complications, the focus of maintenance sessions should be on preventing relapses and addressing them when they occur. Preventing relapses may be accomplished by planning ahead and problem solving. Relapses should be expected, and this should be made clear to parents and children. Families should have an anticipatory strategy for dealing with relapses when they occur. In most cases, this may be just getting "back on" the program—starting to self-monitor again, identifying where the "slips" have occurred, setting short-term behavior change goals, making contracts for changes, monitoring progress, and rewarding success.

References

1. Barlow SE, Dietz WH: Obesity evaluation and treatment: Expert committee recommendations. Pediatrics: 102, 1998. Available at: http//www.pediatrics.org/cgi/content/full/102/3/e29.
2. Robinson TN: Behavioural treatment of childhood and adolescent obesity. Int J Obesity 23(Suppl 2):S52-S57, 1999.
3. Dietz WH, Robinson TN: Use of the body mass index (BMI) as a measure of overweight in children and adolescents. J Pediatr 132:191-93, 1998.
4. Rolland-Cachera M, Deheeger M, Ballisle F, et al: Adiposity rebound in children: a simple indicator for predicting obesity. Am J Clin Nutr 39:129-35, 1984.

ACKNOWLEDGMENT

This work was supported in part by grants from the Children's Health Institute, Department of Pediatrics, Stanford University School of Medicine and the Lucile Packard Children's Hospital at Stanford, and a Robert Wood Johnson Foundation Generalist Physician Faculty Scholar Award.

Chapter 19

Morgan Downey, J.D.

Insurance Coverage for Obesity Treatments

■ Inadequacy of Coverage

It is no secret to primary care providers that reimbursement for obesity treatment is currently one of the great anomalies of the American health care system. Obesity is a serious disease associated with increased mortality rates and an independent cause of hypertension, type-2 diabetes, coronary artery disease, degenerative joint disease, and several types of cancer. These disorders are among the most common, serious, and costly in our society. Yet reimbursement for obesity treatment services is almost nonexistent.

Overweight and obese individuals and the physicians who care for them feel a sense of injustice when health insurers pay for treating complications of obesity like type-2 diabetes, but will not pay for treatments that address the cause, obesity. In addition, many health plans cover other conditions that are not associated with the morbidity or mortality that obesity produces. Medicaid and other health plans cover prescriptions of Viagra for male erectile dysfunction, but do not cover many forms of obesity treatment. Few would argue that male erectile dysfunction is as serious a threat to health as obesity.

Because of this lack of coverage, more people are in need of obesity treatment services than are currently receiving them. For many overweight and obese individuals the costs of services are a substantial deterrent to seeking and receiving treatment. They simply do not have adequate funds to pay for treatment out of pocket and so try to treat themselves with over-the-counter remedies and self-help books. The marketplace appears to be geared to produce obesity and profit on its treatment. Everything that it takes to become overweight seems cheap and plentiful, yet everything it takes to manage weight effectively costs time or money, and usually both. The obese patient gets little support from health insurance institutions.

■ What is Covered?

Medicare, the federal program for health services for the elderly and the disabled, does not consider obesity to be a disease or illness[1] and thus will make no payments for any services in connection with it. In some situations, the Medicare program does recognize gastric bypass surgery[2] as a form of treatment for diabetes or heart disease. Recently, Congress expanded coverage for medical nutrition therapy under Medicare but obesity is not on the list of covered diagnoses. Current legislation under consideration in Congress would expand Medicare by covering drugs for beneficiaries. Weight loss medications are excluded from all of the current proposals.

The Medicaid program, a joint federal–state program for the coverage of the poor and disabled, also does not recognize obesity as a disease. As with Medicare, some states do pay for obesity surgery, although the number of such claims and low reimbursement rates suggest that this benefit is not widely used. The federal statute governing Medicaid coverage of pharmacological compounds specifically excludes payment for drugs for weight loss. However, states can apply for a wavier from this provision. States covering no weight loss drugs include Illinois, Indiana, Nevada, New Hampshire, New York, Ohio, Oklahoma, South Carolina, South Dakota, and Wyoming. States covering orlistat, sibutramine, and phentermine include California, Delaware, Hawaii, Kentucky, Maine, Massachusetts, Mississippi, Montana, New Mexico, Oregon, Rhode Island, Vermont, and Virginia. In some of these states, coverage is conditional on recipients either being morbidly obese or having hyperlipidemia or type-2 diabetes. The remaining states have coverage of less than the three products.

The Child Health Insurance Program, designed to bring more children under Medicaid coverage, does not cover obesity treatments. Other public programs, such as the medical programs of the Veterans Administration, the Indian Health Service, and CHAMPUS, the program of the Department of Defense which covers military personnel and their dependents, do not appear to routinely cover obesity treatments.

Private sector health insurance coverage is not much better. Some managed care companies and Health Maintenance Organizations do provide some support such as corporate wellness programs which incorporate weight management, prescription drugs, reimbursement for membership in weight loss programs, and surgery. Many programs require a comorbid condition such as hyperlipidemia or type-2 diabetes as a condition of covering weight loss treatments. Few companies have shown the leadership of General Motors, which not only covers treatments as part of their health plan but is also working in Flint, Michigan to develop a community-wide approach to healthier living.

■ Why Is Insurance Coverage so Poor?

There are several putative reasons for this lack of coverage. There is a lack of understanding that obesity is a disease and a perception that treatments lack effectiveness. The size of the potential population which would utilize such a benefit threatens high costs, and beliefs about the role of personal responsibility in the etiology of the condition are often skewed.

In contrast to the lack of recognition by insurers, obesity is recognized as a disease by numerous scientific and medical authorities. These include the World Health Organization,[4] the National Academy of Sciences,[3] the National

Institutes of Health,[5] the Food and Drug Administration,[6] the Social Security Administration,[7] the International Classification of Diseases,[8] medical texts, and other authorities. However, the concept of obesity as a disease has yet to gain wide popular acceptance among the public and health care professionals.

There is little doubt that the public and many physicians do not regard weight loss treatments as effective. To some extent, this is a carry-over from previous failures in obesity treatments. This view stems from the unrealistic goals that patients and professionals set for weight-loss treatment programs. To a certain extent, obesity treatments are held to a higher standard of effectiveness than other medical treatments. Many accepted therapies covered by insurance providers fail to produce a complete cure in many cases. For many chronic diseases, treatments are viewed as supportive or palliative and not necessarily curative. Compared to treatments for other lifelong serious conditions or malignancies, obesity treatments demonstrate reasonable effectiveness (see chapter 17 on the National Weight Control Registry and chapter 14 on drug treatment of obesity). While all hope that the effectiveness of treatment modalities will improve over time, questions arise as to what level of effectiveness would be required before coverage would be extended. What criteria would be used to make such a decision? The development of newer, more effective therapies may be slowed by the perception that there will not be coverage for these therapies when they reach the market.

Payers have legitimate concerns about the financial exposure of covering a treatment for which millions of persons would immediately be eligible. This is a real problem that needs to be addressed directly. However, creative and equitable solutions could and should be sought. Financial control could be exercised by reasonable combinations of limitations on the amount or duration of services, patient selection criteria, copayments, and/or caps on annual or lifetime payments.

Beliefs about the role of personal responsibility and weight control are perhaps the most significant obstacles to health-insurance reimbursement. There is a widespread belief that overweight or obese individuals are responsible for their health problem and therefore insurance coverage is not appropriate. While it is true that personal behavior is involved in the genesis of the disorder, this argument has several problems. First, increasing evidence points to a biologic basis for obesity. Second, many health care conditions involve personal behavior. Hypertension, diabetes, sexually transmitted diseases, including HIV/AIDs, and sports injuries all are caused by or are made worse by personal behaviors that do not promote health. Some thirty-percent of all cancers are reportedly due to diet, nutrition, and physical inactivity. Yet no one says "We won't pay for your diabetes or melanoma treatment. You did it yourself." The public and payers seem to see personal behavior as a more important cause of disease when it comes to obesity, an opinion not well supported by relevant science. Treatment costs for many of these conditions are covered by insurance, but obesity treatment costs are not.

■ Signs that Things Are Changing

The situation can improve and has over the last several years. The American Obesity Association (AOA), an advocacy organization, has committed itself to expanding insurance coverage for obesity treatment. Success has been obtained in expanding recognition of obesity as a disease and in working on obtaining reimbursement.

Under previous Internal Revenue Service (IRS) regulations, expenses for weight loss could not be taken as medical-expense deductions. Earlier instructions to taxpayers had stated, "You cannot deduct the cost of weight loss treatment even if your doctor prescribes it."[9] In August of 1999, the AOA put together a coalition of organizations in a petition to the IRS to change this interpretation of the Internal Revenue Code. A year later, the IRS changed its instructions to read, "You can include in medical expense the cost of weight loss program undertaken at a physician's direction to treat an existing disease (such as heart disease). But you cannot include the cost of a weight-loss program if the purpose of the weight control is to maintain your good health."[10]

Subsequently, the AOA asked the Internal Revenue Service for a letter of public information as to whether treatment for obesity (defined as a Body Mass Index $>30kg/M^2$) alone qualified for the deduction. The IRS responded on June 1, 2001. In their response, the IRS stated, "we are aware that there is considerable scientific and regulatory authority that obesity is, in and of itself, a disease. . . . If obesity is a disease, then expenses for the diagnosis and treatment of obesity may qualify as expenses for medical expense. There are, however, certain limitations on the medical expense deduction that may apply to expenses for treating obesity. Expenses for medicines and drugs to assist in weight loss can be for medical care only if the medicine or drug is a prescribed drug or insulin. . . . Additionally, while many obese individuals may follow special diets as part of their treatment, the cost of food is not an expense for medical care to the extent the food is a substitute for the food that an individual would normally consume to meet nutritional requirements. If a special diet is directed as treatment for a disease, only the excess cost of the special diet over the cost of a regular diet could be an expense for medical care." This IRS decision applies not only to individuals who itemize their deductions, but also applies to employees who participate in a medical savings account.

Both the Social Security Administration and the Food and Drug Administration now acknowledge obesity as a disease as a qualifying condition for disability and in regards to advertising restrictions on dietary supplements promoted as weight loss aids.[6,7]

The AOA has initiated a liaison with the American Association of Health Plans, the trade association for the managed care industry, to promote greater coverage of obesity treatment. The AOA continues to actively lobby Congress and the Executive Branch to include obesity treatment in the Medicare drug benefit proposals. The AOA has also distributed over two million brochures, *Weight Management and Health Insurance* to empower individuals to advocate with their employers for improved coverage.

In April 2001, the Centers for Disease Control and Prevention held a two-day workshop in Atlanta, GA on reimbursement for obesity treatment. A steering committee was formed and this group has begun an effort to develop a coalition of organizations that will provide ongoing leadership in this area.

■ What You and Your Patients Can Do

Individual physicians, other health care providers and their patients and families need to be proactive in obtaining improved reimbursement. Physicians should encourage patients to file for health-insurance coverage for obesity. If the claims are rejected, appeals should be filed. Patients should be encouraged to talk with their employers about including coverage. If the patients are not comfortable doing this, they should be encouraged to ask a coworker to be their advocate. Health care professionals should also take opportunities such as health fairs and meetings with state and federal elected officials to communicate the true picture of the obesity epidemic in the country and the need for treatment. Local and state medical societies and professional and business groups should be encouraged to take positions in support of obesity treatments.

In such efforts, confidence and persistence count. The health care system is paying millions of dollars treating disorders that could be prevented or ameliorated by sustained weight loss. The growing epidemic of obesity among children and adolescents means more potentially preventable morbidity and mortality in years to come, not to mention potentially avoidable health care expenditures. Advocates should insist that obesity be considered with the same standards used to make coverage decisions for other diseases. It is a form of discrimination to hold obesity treatment to standards that are not applied to other conditions. For example, payers sometimes want to see tangible proof that coverage of obesity treatments will save them money. However, they do not apply this standard to other therapeutic areas. Another strategy used by payers is to "condition coverage" of obesity treatments on the presence of type-2 diabetes or heart disease. This "cueing" is not wise health policy as it does not allow the benefits of obesity treatment used to prevent disease, and it is not used for other conditions. Treatment for diabetes is not withheld until complications develop.

Clearly, issues of treatment effectiveness, cost of treatment, and which patients should be covered need to be addressed directly with an open and frank discussion of what standards are reasonable and appropriate. Always go through proper channels within insurance or managed care companies, e.g., customer services, director of customer services, marketing director. The medical director is a key individual in making coverage decisions. Patients who have medical savings accounts should be encouraged to put aside pre-tax dollars into such accounts for future employee expenses. Collect helpful supporting information. The NIH/NIHLBI Guidelines for the treatment of Adult Obesity can be very useful in demonstrating the acceptance and effectiveness of obesity treatment. The AOA website, www.obesity.org, is also a resouce of materials useful for these efforts (see chapter 20 for other useful web resources).

The situation will change. The obesity epidemic is simply too large to be ignored for much longer. New treatments are being developed. New studies are demonstrating the effectiveness of many forms of intervention. Professionals have a duty not only to be well informed about their patients and their disease and treatments; they have a duty to advocate for those who need help. Finally, presumably large numbers of persons with obesity have no health insurance at all. Expanding insurance programs to cover more persons without any coverage is also vitally important.

References

1. Health Care Financing Administration Coverage Issues Manual ¶35-26.
2. Health Care Financing Administration Coverage Issues Manual ¶ 35-40.
3. Weighing the Options, Criteria for Evaluating Weight Management Programs, Paul R. Thomas, Editor, Institute of Medicine, National Academy Press, Washington, DC, 1995.
4. WHO Press Release 46, 12 June 1997.
5. Clinical Guidelines on the Identification, Evaluation, and Treatment of Overweight and Obesity in Adults, The Evidence Report, National Institutes of Health, National Heart, Lung and Blood Institute, No. 98-4083, 1998.
6. Federal Register, January 6, 2000, Vol. 65, p. 1028.
7. Federal Register, Vol. 65, No. 94, May 15, 2000, p. 31039.
8. The ICD-9-CM lists "Obesity and other hyperalimentation" as #278 in the Endocrine, Nutritional, Metabolic and Immunity Disorders section.
9. IRS Publication 502 for 1999 tax year.
10. IRS Publication 502 for 2000 tax year.

Chapter 20

Laura E. Primak, RD, CSP, CNSD

Obesity Web Resources for Health Professionals

The Internet boasts a wealth of information. Both patients and health professionals are turning to this source for facts, answers, and advice. Nutrition, diet, and exercise information are contained on literally thousands of web sites. Overweight and obesity are topics that over half of all Americans are struggling with, and the Internet offers quick information on support and solutions. For health professionals, the Internet can offer a convenient and quick way to get current information on obesity research, obesity treatments, and trends in obesity management and care.

However, the validity of information on many Internet sites is often questionable. There are a large number of sites that are designed to make money first and provide information second. The old admonition "buyer beware" applies. Fortunately, there are many sites that provide reliable information. This chapter briefly reviews how to know when a site is worthy of spending time and provides a list of Internet resources covering a wide range of obesity related issues.

The most important factor in determining the reliability of the information presented on a web site is the source. Who is providing the site and what is the motivation behind the information? Educational? Academic? Selling a product? Making a profit? Most reputable web sites on obesity come from academic, research, professional, and government sources. Some may provide publications and other products for a fee, but they exist primarily to educate the public and/or health professionals. Web sites sponsored by companies (e.g., pharmaceutical companies, etc.) can still provide worthwhile information, but the source should be kept in mind.

Other factors helping determine the usefulness of a given site are ease of navigation, clarity of information provided, and the provision of scientific and evidence-based information with references available to support claims or data provided.

When armed with well-developed and informative sites, health professionals can find the Internet to be one of their most valuable tools for patient care issues and professional growth.

■ General Obesity Information

National Heart Lung and Blood Institute

This organization provides excellent information on cardiovascular diseases as well as obesity topics for health professionals and for patients.

http://www.nhlbi.nih.gov/guidelines/obesity/ob_home.htm—Federal clinical guidelines for the identification, evaluation, and treatment of overweight and obesity in adults. Several different formats of this comprehensive report are available for viewing on this site.

National Institute for Diabetes, Digestive, and Kidney Diseases

The NIDDK is the primary research organization for obesity of the National Institute of Health. The site provides information on a variety of health topics as well as research funding opportunities, clinical trials, health education programs, and special reports.

http://www.niddk.nih.gov/health/nutrit/win.htm—The Weight Information Network was established in 1994 to provide health professionals and consumers with science-based information on obesity, weight control, and nutrition. Includes a variety of publications, brochures, a free newsletter, and research information.

http://www.niddk.nih.gov/health/nutrit/pubs/statobes.htm—Statistics related to overweight and obesity, including statistics on prevalence and economic costs of these conditions.

National Library of Medicine

http://www.nlm.nih.gov/medlineplus/obesity.html—Medline Plus Health Information provides a multitude of information and links for obesity from the latest news on obesity, recent research articles, general information, nutrition and treatment information, and clinical trials.

http://text.nlm.nih.gov/cps/www/cps.27.html—Literature review discussing the prevalence of overweight and obesity, risk factors, and observational study data establishing a clear association between overweight and hypercholesterolemia are presented. Recommendations of the American Academy of Family Physicians, the American Heart Association, the American Medical Association, and other reputable sources are included.

American Association of Clinical Endocrinologists

http://www.aace.com/clin/guidelines/obesityguide.pdf—This position paper on obesity is a first-class resource. The result of an expert review, this detailed and referenced position paper expresses the cutting edge of medical opinion on the causes, diagnosis, and management of obesity as of 1998 (Adobe Acrobat reader is required to view this document).

Arborcom.com

http://arborcom.com/frame/wtloss.htm—"Managing the overweight patient"—a brief but excellent article written for family physicians on this challenging issue.

Heart Information Network

http://www.heartinfo.com/search/display.asp?id=455—The library section features a variety of articles summarizing recent research findings related to adult and pediatric obesity, nutrition, and fitness and their application to clinical care.

Merck Manual of Diagnosis and Therapy

http://www.merck.com/pubs/mmanual/section1/chapter5/5a.htm—Thorough chapter discussing the epidemiology, etiology, complications, and treatment of obesity.

■ Pediatric Obesity

Pediatrics (Journal)

http://www.pediatrics.org/cgi/reprint/102/3/e29.pdf—"Obesity Evaluation and Treatment: Expert Committee Recommendations Practice Guidelines" for practitioners who evaluate and treat overweight children. (Adobe Acrobat Reader is necessary to access this document.). A must read for those caring for overweight/obese pediatric patients.

National Academy Press

http://www.nap.edu/catalog/4756.html—"Weighing the Options: Criteria for Evaluating Weight-Management Programs." Paul R. Thomas, Editor; Committee to Develop Criteria for Evaluating the Outcomes of Approaches to Prevent and Treat Obesity, Institute of Medicine 1995. Read it free online. Appendix C covers childhood obesity and is an excellent text overview of the multi-faceted problems of this disorder.

United States Department of Agriculture

http://www.usda.gov/cnpp/Seminars/obesity.PDF—Childhood Obesity, Causes and Treatments 1998 symposium proceedings by the Center for Nutrition Policy and Promotion. Includes a series of presentations and discussions. Requires Adobe Acrobat Reader to open file. Good information.

American Heart Association

http://www.americanheart.org/Scientific/statements/1996/1202.html—Medical/scientific statement on understanding obesity in youth by the American Heart Association. No frills but excellent information.

Child Obesity

http://www.childobesity.com/—This site provides resources on child obesity for health professionals, educators, and families. There is good background information on pediatric obesity with multiple assessment tools, educational programs, and training materials that can be ordered. The majority of the materials were developed at the University of California San Francisco.

■ Treatment Information

General

Partnership for Healthy Weight Management

http://www.consumer.gov/weightloss/—The Partnership for Healthy Weight Management is a coalition of representatives from science, academia, the health care profession, government, commercial enterprises, and organizations whose mission is to promote sound guidance on strategies for achieving and maintaining a healthy weight.

Weight Management through Lifestyle

http://www.mayohealth.org/home?id=SP4.1.5.6 - A collection of weight management articles from the MayoClinic.com website.

Federal Trade Commission/Skinny on Dieting

http://www.ftc.gov/bcp/conline/pubs/health/diets.htm - A brief article by the Federal Trade Commission that focuses on deceptive diet advertisements and how to tell the realistic programs from the unrealistic. Also provides some interesting dieting statistics.

HealthAtoZ.com

http://216.255.140.184/atoz/obesity/treat.html—Overview of obesity treatments including some information on herbal and over-the-counter treatments.

Michael D. Myers, MD, Inc.

http://www.weight.com/—The information on this site is provided by Michael D. Myers, MD, Inc. who states "the purpose of this site is to provide objective medical information on obesity, eating disorders, and associated medical conditions in a non-commercial environment where any editorial comment is appropriately noted." He is a practicing physician, member of NAASO (North American Association for the Study of Obesity) who has actively treated obesity and (to a lesser extent) eating disorders for over 17 years. This site provides good information on a variety of obesity related topics.

Medications

National Institute of Diabetes, Digestive, and Kidney Diseases

http://www.niddk.nih.gov/health/nutrit/pubs/presmeds.htm—A nice overview of prescription medications used in the treatment of obesity sponsored by the Weight Information Network.

Roche Pharmaceuticals

http://www.rocheusa.com/products/xenical/pi.html—Xenical product information from Roche Pharmaceuticals. Includes information on clinical pharmacology and clinical studies, as well as dosing information.

Knoll Pharmaceuticals

http://www.4meridia.com/hcprof/fin.htm—All about Meridia from Knoll Pharmaceuticals, including mechanism of action, safety, behavioral changes, side effects, efficacy, and prescribing information.

Surgery

American Society for Bariatric Surgery

http://www.asbs.org/html/ration.html—This site provides excellent information on the pros and cons of bariatric surgery, as well as the nutritional consequences of surgery, patient selection criteria, and psychological issues.

Exercise and Physical Activity

Centers for Disease Control

http://www.cdc.gov/nccdphp/dnpa/—The National Center for Disease Control and Health Prevention's web site on nutrition and physical activity. Contains information on prevalence of obesity and physical inactivity, public health programs, press releases, and training and software tools. Easy to navigate with good information.

Shape Up America!

http://www.shapeup.org/—This website is designed to provide the latest information about safe weight management, healthy eating, increased activity, and physical fitness. Good information and fun tools.

http://www.shapeup.org/professional/index.html—This site allows access to the "Guidance for the Treatment of Adult Obesity" publication. Adobe Acrobat Reader is needed to view the documents.

American College of Sports Medicine

http://www.acsm.org/—The mission of the ACSM is to promote and integrate scientific research, education, and practical applications of sports medicine and exercise science to maintain and enhance physical performance, fitness, health, and quality of life. While much of this site is geared toward members, good information can still be found.

American Council on Exercise

http://www.acefitness.org/—The "Fit Facts" section provides many good articles on a variety of exercise and fitness issues.

Dr. Koop's Health Site

http://www.drkoop.com/dyncon/center.asp?id=1036—Dr. Koop's (former Surgeon General) Fitness Center provides a variety of interesting information on activity, from smart summer workouts to muscle pain management to fitness facts and more. Though aimed more at the general population, it is still a great resource for the public and health professionals.

Food and Nutrition

The American Dietetic Association
http://www.eatright.org—This site provides a variety of information on nutrition and health, has a search engine allowing topic searches, and provides a way to locate dietitians across the U.S. This is a good site to start any search for nutrition topics.

Nutrition.gov
http://www.nutrition.gov—A guide to nutrition and health information on government web sites. A huge site with lots to offer, but best to have a specific topic or area in mind when setting out on a search, or the volume of information available could easily be overwhelming.

USDA

Food and Nutrition Information Center
http://www.nal.usda.gov/fnic/Fpyr/pyramid.html—Information about the Food Guide Pyramid and how it can be used with different populations (pediatric, ethnic, etc.). The site is easy to use and provides a good resource on healthy eating materials.

Nutrient Data Laboratory
http://www.nal.usda.gov/fnic/foodcomp/,Use this site to search their nutrient database, look up food sources of vitamin K, or see which foods have oxalic acid, and a host of other interesting information about nutrients and foods.

Dietary Guidelines for Americans
http://www.health.gov/dietaryguidelines/—The USDA periodically updates the Dietary Guidelines for Americans that focus on physical activity and eating a variety of foods, especially vegetables, fruits, and whole grains.

Obesity Medical Associations

North American Society for the Study of Obesity
http://www.naaso.org/— The North American Association for the Study of Obesity is the premier scientific society for scientists whose research focuses on biology related to the clinical problem of obesity. It is an interdisciplinary society whose purpose is to develop, extend, and disseminate knowledge in the field of obesity. The site provides information on membership, meetings and conferences, news/press releases, and access to the official journal of NAASO—Obesity Research. Note that the discussion group feature is available to members only.

International Obesity Task Force (IOTF)

http://www.iotf.org—Part of the International Association for the Study of Obesity (IASO) which is the premier international scientific society for scientists and professionals studying the problem of obesity. IOTF has been charged with alerting the world of the growing health crisis from the soaring levels of obesity. This site provides international obesity information and has a variety of publications.

American Obesity Association

http://www.obesity.org—This is a relatively new organization whose mission is educating the public about obesity and its role in causing illness and unnecessary deaths, and helping health professionals to provide the best possible care for people with obesity. This site provides very good information on obesity treatments, medical conditions associated with obesity, and general obesity information.

American Society of Bariatric Physicians

http://www.asbp.org—A national professional medical specialty society of licensed physicians who offer specialized programs in the medical treatment of obesity and its associated conditions. This organization is not formally affiliated with the more mainstream and scientifically-based NASSO. This organization is largely an association of clinical practitioners who have defined themselves as experts in obesity treatment. ASBP offers continuing medical education programs, a uarterly journal, The American Journal of Bariatric Medicine—The Bariatrician, and a bi-monthly newsletter, News from ASBP. While many practitioners who participate in ASBP are excellent, the lack of a research focus in the organization and the commercial emphasis of some of the members is concerning to some obesity professionals.

■ Research Centers

Boston Obesity and Nutrition Research Center

http://www.bmc.org/bonrc/—The Boston Obesity Nutrition Research Center (BONRC) is an inter-institutional unit with an overall goal to understand the etiology of and find effective treatment for obesity and related disorders, and to educate and train investigators in these areas.

Center for Obesity Research and Education

http://www.uchsc.edu/core—The Centers for Obesity Research and Education (C.O.R.E.) was formed in 1998 to provide guidance and training for health care providers on how to manage their obese patients.

Minnesota Obesity and Nutrition Research Center

http://www.umn.edu/mnoc—The Minnesota Obesity Center is an Obesity Nutrition Research Center (ONRC) funded by the National Institute of

Diabetes and Digestive and Kidney Diseases (NIDDK) of the National Institutes of Health. The mission of the Minnesota Obesity Center is to find ways
to prevent weight gain, obesity, and its complications.

New York Obesity and Nutrition Research Center
http://www.niddk.nih.gov/fund/other/centers/newyork.htm—The New
York Obesity/Nutrition Research Center (ONRC) was established in 1979
and is funded by the National Institute of Diabetes and Digestive and Kidney Diseases (NIDDK). Primary research efforts are in the areas of obesity
genetics, measurement of body composition, and the effects of central body
fat distribution in relation to health risks.

Pittsburgh Obesity and Nutrition Research Center
http://www.wpic.pitt.edu/onrc—The University of Pittsburgh Obesity/
Nutrition Research Center (ONRC) was established in 1992 with funding
from the National Institute of Diabetes and Digestive and Kidney Diseases.
The University of Pittsburgh ONRC focuses on behavioral aspects of obesity and behavioral treatment of this disease.

■ On-line Journals and Newsletters

Obesity Research
http://www.obesityresearch.org/—The official journal of the North
American Association for the Study of Obesity. This peer-reviewed journal
offers the latest research on obesity.

International Journal of Obesity
http://www.naturesj.com/ijo/index.html—The audience for this journal
includes clinicians and researchers working in obesity, diabetes and related
disorders, dietetics, psychology, psychiatry, epidemiology, metabolic function, biochemistry, physiology, molecular biology, and genetics.

Obesity Reviews
http://www.blackwell-synergy.com/Journals/issuelist.asp?journal=obr—
Official journal of the International Association for the Study of Obesity. It is
a vehicle for publishing updated reviews in all disciplines related to obesity.

Obesity Surgery
http://www.obesitysurgery.com/—The official journal for the American
Society of Bariatric Surgeons. This journal provides an international and
interdisciplinary forum for communicating the latest research and surgical
techniques in Bariatric surgery.

■ Patient Education Materials

American Dietetic Association
Nutrition Fact Sheets
http://www.eatright.org/nfs/ - This collection of nutrition fact sheets covers everything from weight management to vegetarian eating to healthy child nutrition. A great collection and resource.

National Heart Lung and Blood Institute
http://www.nhlbi.nih.gov/health/pubs/pub_gen.htm#obesity—The NHLBI has many good publications for patients on obesity and fitness.

National Institute of Diabetes, Digestive, and Kidney Diseases
http://www.niddk.nih.gov/health/nutrit/pubs/choose.htm—This information is provided by the Weight Control Information Network, and offers sound advice about the approach to weight loss and evaluating programs based on safety, efficacy, and each individual's needs. By clicking on the "publications" link a variety of other materials written primarily for the public on weight loss and control can be seen.

Federal Consumer Information Center
http://www.pueblo.gsa.gov/food.htm—Provides a list of brochures and materials on a variety of nutrition topics that can be obtained for free or read on-line.

Food and Health Communications
http://www.foodandhealth.com/handout.shtml—This site offers a handful of free nutrition handouts on topics such as weight loss and why low carbohydrate diets may be harmful for health. Limited variety, but what they have is good.

Interactive Healthy Eating Index
http://63.73.158.75/—This interactive tool allows the visitor to enter 1-20 days of diet intake information and have it analyzed for the quality of the diet and a comparison to the food guide pyramid. Site does require that you register with them in order to use the features.

American Academy of Family Physicians
http://familydoctor.org/cgi-bin/list.pl?element=handout—An extensive collection of over 300 handouts on a variety of medical conditions and issues. You have to search a bit, but there are handouts on nutrition, weight loss, and fitness. This is a nice resource for professionals.

■ Conclusion

While these listings are by no means comprehensive they will offer a good start. Many of these sites have links to other related sites. Of course some sites are better than others, and this chapter places particularly excellent sites at the top of these lists. This is not to say that there are not other excellent sites on the web. *Happy Surfing*.

Chapter 21

Daniel H. Bessesen, MD

Regulation of Appetite by the Central Nervous System

When discussing a weight management program with a patient, it can be challenging to balance the need to encourage them to have a sense of hope that the weight loss program will succeed versus the reality that losing weight for many people is an extremely difficult task. They may have feelings that their body weight is the product of a "weak will" or "bad behaviors." It may be useful to tell them that the regulation of body weight is a complicated biologic process which has evolved over many thousands of years. The behaviors needed to acquire food are some of the most complex and potentially risky that any organism engages in. It may be useful to remind the patient that the drive to find and eat food evolved in an environment where food was scarce and getting adequate nutrition required a great deal of effort. Suggest that "being overweight is not something that you've chosen," or "think of the weight problem much the same way as high blood pressure, blood glucose, or cholesterol levels—it is a chronic metabolic problem that is in part biologic." This can help remove fault or guilt over a weight problem. There are complex systems within the brain that cause a person to feel hunger, consume nutrients, and expend energy.

This review will provide an overview of some of what has been learned over the last ten years about the neural systems that regulate body weight. There has been an explosion of knowledge about the neuropeptides that regulate appetite and body weight, which has been the result of applying modern molecular techniques to the study of rodent models of obesity. There are a number of strains of mice and rats that transmit obesity in a manner consistent with a single gene defect. Over the last ten years a number of the genes that produce obesity in these mice have been identified and we are beginning to gain an understanding of how these peptides function.

■ Overview of Neurotransmitter Systems

There are essentially three categories of neurotransmitters. The first is gamma-aminobutyric acid (GABA). GABA functions throughout the central nervous system essentially as an on/off switch that turns on a variety of neural circuits. Its function is critical for maintaining a state of arousal, but its effects are not specific for any particular system or behavior. The second category of neurotransmitters are the monoamines. These include the neurotransmitters norepinephrine, dopamine, and serotonin. These neurotransmitters are widely distributed through the nervous system and function in some ways as a "volume control" on a variety of systems, turning pathways up or down. These neurotransmitters do not produce effects on specific behaviors but instead have effects on a variety of systems and behaviors. Dopamine appears to be important in reward characteristics of feeding, but does not seem to be directly involved in appetite per say. Norepinephrine and serotonin appear to have important effects on the regulation of body weight. These two transmitters are present in a number of brain centers within the hypothalamus that are involved in eating and body weight regulation. These transmitter systems are the targets of currently available medications,which have shown some effectiveness in altering body weight including phentermine, sibutramine, and the previously available fenfluramine and dexfenfluramine. The effects of these two transmitters extend beyond feeding behavior to other systems including autonomic regulation and mood. Additionally, these neurotransmitters have a complex physiology, including multiple receptor subtypes and regulated reuptake from the nerve terminals that release them.

Neuropeptides are the third class of neurotransmitters. They have the most specific effects on individual behaviors and body functions. While there are a large number of neuropeptides, each having associated complexities in receptor subtypes and interactions with other neural circuits, it is hoped that drug targets within the neuropeptide systems may prove effective in altering body weight without other unwanted side effects. Much of our recent understanding of the specific neuropeptides which regulate body weight have come from the cloning of genes that cause obesity in monogenic rodent models of obesity. While the norepinephrine and serotonin systems continue to be a focus of research, it is hoped that neuropeptides systems will provide the specificity to appetite and body weight regulation which seem to be lacking with the monoamine neurotransmitters.

■ Leptin

One of the single-gene models of obesity in mice is the ob/ob mouse. In the 1960's, studies were done using ob/ob mice and the technique of parabiosis. Parabiosis involves connecting two mice together surgically in a manner whereby they do not share blood supplies, but hormones and small molecules can pass from one animal to the other. If a mouse is made obese by virtually any means (overfeeding, hypothalamic lesioning) and it is parabiosed to another mouse, the normal weight partner will gradually reduce its food intake and lose weight. This experimental result suggests that there is a hormone within the obese animal that causes the partner to stop eating. However, if an ob/ob mouse is parabiosed to a normal mouse, the opposite was seen, the ob/ob mouse loses weight. This result was taken as evidence that the ob/ob mouse lacked this weight-regulating hormone. It took more than thirty years for the nature of this substance to be identified, and in 1994, the gene product which was responsible for the obesity in this mouse was cloned. The substance is a hormone secreted by adipose tissue which is not produced in the ob/ob mouse because of a gene mutation. This hormone was given the name leptin after the Greek root *leptos*, which means thin. When recombinant leptin is given to an ob/ob mouse the animal increases its physical activity, reduces its food intake, and loses fat mass specifically with minimal or no loss of lean mass. Leptin was hoped to be a potential "cure for obesity" in humans. However, while human adipose tissue does indeed make leptin, obese humans are not deficient in the hormone, instead they produce increased levels of it. This finding suggests that human obesity is not due to leptin deficiency but rather leptin resistance. Over the next few years a large number of investigators examined the mechanisms by which leptin exerts its effects.

The first step in this process was the identification and cloning of the family of leptin receptors (which some have called obRs). Leptin receptors are produced in a long form and several short forms. The long form of the leptin receptor has an extracellular hormone binding domain, a membrane-spanning sequence, and an intracellular signaling sequence. The sequence of the long form of the leptin receptor is related to cytokine receptors and it makes use of JAK/stat proteins for intracellular signaling. There are also several short forms of the leptin receptor, which do not appear to have the complete intracellular signaling sequence. The long form of the leptin receptor is present in the hypothalamus as well as a number of other extra-hypothalamic brain regions including the hippocampus and cerebellum. The short forms of the leptin receptor are expressed in many tissues, but appear to be particularly important in the choroid plexus where they may function to facilitate transport of leptin from the bloodstream into the brain, the principal site of hormone action. Available evidence suggests that at least part of the resistance to leptin seen in obese humans and diet-induced obesity in rodents is due to a defect in the movement of leptin from the bloodstream into the central nervous system. However, there is increasing evidence that there may also be resistance to the actions of leptin at a post-receptor level.

Leptin, acting through its receptor, has a large number of effects in the brain and in peripheral tissues. Hypothalamic cells exposed to leptin increase the transcription of at least 80 different genes. The result of this activity is a change in neurotransmitter production and cell firing in leptin-responsive cells. In addition, administration of recombinant leptin into the brain of rodents has been shown to alter liver glucose production. Finally, peripheral leptin appears to alter fat metabolism in a number of tissues including skeletal muscle, liver, and pancreatic beta cells. Currently it is not clear whether peripheral effects of leptin on fuel metabolism are primarily due to direct effects of the hormone on skeletal muscle, liver, and pancreas, or secondary to the effects of leptin on neural targets in the brain. The important role of leptin in regulating glucose metabolism has been highlighted recently by the finding that severe insulin resistance present in humans with generalized lipodystrophy can be reversed by administration of recombinant human leptin.

Leptin deficiency has been identified in several obese humans, and in these individuals leptin treatment produced weight loss. It was hoped that recombinant human leptin might be a useful therapeutic agent in the treatment of human obesity. Two companies, Amgen and Roche, have conducted studies in humans of recombinant leptin, but to date these studies have demonstrated that this hormone appears to have a minimal weight-loss effect in most obese humans. It remains unclear what the role of leptin will be in the treatment of obese humans. However, the discovery of leptin and its central-signaling pathways have opened the door to our understanding of central neural pathways involved in the regulation of body weight. These new insights may ultimately lead to the identification of effective treatments even if leptin itself is not found to be that treatment.

■ Neuropeptide Y

Neuropeptide Y (NPY) is a hypothalamic neurotransmitter that is the most potent orexigenic (stimulates food intake) peptide known. In animals that have been fasted, the expression of NPY increases in the hypothalamus, and chronic injections within the central nervous system can produce obesity by overeating. Central administration of NPY, like leptin, appears to alter not only appetite but peripheral metabolism as well. Specifically, central administration of NPY increases fat storage through alterations in adipose tissue lipoprotein lipase and decreases in energy expenditure. This peptide apparently has a broad range of biologic effects that promote weight gain. The level of NPY expression has been found to be increased in a number of rodent models of obesity, suggesting it may play a pathogenic role.

NPY exerts its biologic actions through its own family of receptors. To date, five types of NPY receptors have been identified. These have been named Y1–Y5, with Y1 and Y5 receptor subtypes thought to be the most important in body-weight regulation. NPY is expressed in cells that also express the long form of the leptin receptor. These cells are located in a part of the hypothalamus (the arcuate nucleus) and appear to respond to leptin stimulation by alterations in NPY production. This suggests that NPY cells are downstream effectors of leptin action. Evidence in support of this has come from the observation that ob/ob mice (leptin deficient) have increased levels of NPY expression, yet central administration of leptin decreases NPY expression. It is hoped that drugs which antagonized NPY action at its receptor might be useful therapeutic agents for weight loss drugs. However, to date drugs with this mechanism of action have not shown much efficacy in producing weight loss in animal studies. It seems highly likely that the neural systems which control body weight are redundant and that effective therapy will require drugs which interact with these pathways at multiple points.

■ Melanocortins

Another monogenic rodent model of obesity is the agouti mouse (ay/ay). This mouse (named for its gold coat) is obese and insulin resistant. Using modern molecular techniques, the abnormal gene responsible for the phenotype of this mouse strain was identified. The alterations in color and weight are due to the overexpression of a peptide named agouti protein by the skin. This protein is an antagonist of the melanocortin receptors. Melanocortins are a class of hormones that include agouti protein, malanocyte-stimulating hormones (MSH), and agouti-related peptide (AGRP). The melanocortin that is most familiar is alpha MSH. This hormone is a fragment of the larger pro-opiomelanocortin or POMC gene product that is made by the anterior pituitary. POMC is also the precursor for adrenocorticotropic hormone (ACTH). ACTH regulates steroid production by the adrenal glands and MSH regulates among other things skin pigmentation. MSH binds to a family of receptors known as the melanocortin receptors. Currently, five melanocortin receptors have been identified. Activation of the MC1 receptor appears to be important in coat color through inducing pigment production by the hair follicle. The MC4 and MC3 receptors are important in body weight regulation. Evidence of the importance of the MC4 receptor in body weight regulation comes from studies of mice that have had this receptor knocked out. These mice are obese and insulin resistant. Stimulation of the MC4 receptor by MSH or other ligands reduces food intake. Several humans have been identified with MC4 mutations who have red hair, are fair skinned, and are also obese. Another example of the importance of endogenous alpha MSH in regulating body weight is apparent from the POMC knockout mouse, which lacks alpha MSH, overeats, and is obese. This suggests that endogenous alpha MSH is an agonist of MC4 receptors, and its absence causes obesity. The MC2 receptor is expressed in the adrenal cortex and allows the adrenal gland to respond to ACTH. The MC5 receptor is expressed in sebaceous glands and is involved in temperature regulation.

Another way to decrease signaling along this pathway besides knocking out the receptor is through antagonism at the receptor. The agouti mouse makes a protein that functions in this manner. This protein is usually not made in peripheral tissues, but in the agouti mouse it is. The result is a reduction in fur pigmentation, increased food intake, and obesity, due to antagonism with the MC4 receptor. Although this mouse model of obesity provided the first clue of the importance of melanocortins in body weight regulation, to date no cases of human obesity have been identified that are due to ectopic production of agouti protein.

The melanocortin pathway that regulates body weight is even more complex. There exists an endogenous antagonist produced within the hypothalamus named agouti-related peptide or AGRP. AGRP is an endogenous antagonist of the melanocortin pathway that acts as a long-acting stimulator of food intake. The agonist MSH and the antagonist AGRP stimulate or inhibit the function of the MC4 receptor. It appears that this system functions downstream of leptin, since animals without MC4 receptors do not respond to leptin. Cells expressing MC4 receptors are present in the arcuate nucleus of the hypothalamus. Since recent studies in humans have demonstrated limited effectiveness of leptin as a weight loss treatment, several drug companies have shifted their focus to the melanocortin system in their search for drug targets that might prove to be useful in the treatment of obese humans. The strategy has been to use the predicted structure of the MC4 receptor to try to design orally administered MC4 agonists that might inhibit appetite.

■ Mahogany

Another single gene rodent model of obesity was given the name Mahogany because of its hair color. Mahogany mice are of normal body weight and, when bred with agouti (ay) mice, the offspring do not have the golden color or obesity typical of that strain. This was the first evidence that this gene is important in the regulation of body weight and that it likely interacts somehow with the melanocortin pathway. Mahogany mice who are fed a high-fat diet do not become obese as other strains of mice typically do, suggesting that this gene is also important in regulating body weight in the setting of a highly palatable diet. This gene has been cloned and the structure suggests a single transmembrane protein. This peptide appears to be expressed in a number of brain regions outside the hypothalamus. Much needs to be learned about the function of this protein and how it interacts with the melanocortin system to regulate body weight. At this time understanding of its function is so preliminary that it does not appear to be a target for weight-loss drugs.

■ Orexin A/B

With the advent of molecular cloning techniques, a large number of novel gene products have been identified whose function is not yet known. One approach to identifying the function of these genes is to look for structural similarities between the novel gene and genes whose products have known functions. This strategy was used by a group at Southwestern University to identify the function of several gene products that resemble known g-coupled receptors. These genes, known as orphan receptors, have been known for some time now. What the researchers did was to use a novel expression cloning strategy whereby cells that were designed to produce these putative receptors were exposed to proteins produced by other unidentified genes isolated from mRNAs produced by the brain. They measured the production of cyclic AMP, which told them that the unknown peptide was a ligand for the unknown receptor.

Using this strategy the researchers identified two ligands known as orexin A and orexin B, and the two associated receptors that bind these neuropeptides. Administration of recombinant orexin into the hypothalamus of rats stimulates feeding behavior. Expression of orexin in the hypothalamus increases in fasted animals. In an attempt to establish the role of orexin in body weight regulation, mice were generated with orexin A and B knocked out. The unexpected finding was that these mice had narcolepsy. Since that initial discovery, it has been found that some dogs and humans afflicted with narcolepsy have mutations in the orexin gene. Orexin is expressed in cells of the lateral hypothalamus consistent with the hypothesis that this brain region might be a "feeding center." Studies demonstrate that orexin expression is modulated by leptin signals within the hypothalamus. To date no studies have been published using drugs that interact as antagonists with these receptors, and the relative importance of orexins as compared to other neuropeptides in the regulation of body weight is not clear.

■ Cocaine Amphetamine Related Transcript (CART)

Another recently discovered gene product that appears to be important in regulating food intake and body weight is cocaine amphetamine related transcript (CART). This gene product was cloned from the central nervous system of rats that were chronically exposed to cocaine. A subtraction cloning strategy was used to identify novel genes expressed in the brains of cocaine-addicted animals. When this gene product was identified and recombinant protein injected into rats, the animals reduced their food intake. CART is expressed by cells in the arcuate nucleus of the hypothalamus. Its expression in the hypothalamus decreases with fasting and increases with peripheral leptin injection. The mRNA for this gene is reduced or absent in ob/ob mice which suggest that cells which produce CART are downstream of the leptin responsive cells. To date the structure of the receptor for this peptide is not known, and there are no drugs that interact directly with this system. However, since this an anorectic pathway, there may be hope for future medications which act on this system.

■ Melanin-Concentrating Hormone

Melanin-concentrating hormone (MCH) is a hormone secreted by the pituitary gland. It was first identified many years ago by its ability to cause changes in the coloring of fish scales. It does this by inducing a migration of pigment-producing cells into the scale. Its role in body weight regulation was identified more recently through a subtraction cloning strategy that was used to identify genes that were differentially expressed in obese ob/ob mice as compared to lean mice. It was discovered that obese mice had increased expression of MCH. Once this observation was made, recombinant MCH was produced and injected into the third ventricle of rats. MCH stimulated food intake in these animals. MCH is expressed in the lateral hypothalamus, and MCH knockout mice are anorectic and lean. The structures of two MCH receptors have recently been published. These were named SRC-1 and MCHr. These receptors appear to be coupled to g-proteins. Already there are drug development programs targeting compounds that act as antagonists to these receptors

TABLE 1. Neuropeptides Regulating Feeding

Orexigenic	Anorexigenic
NPY	alpha MSH
AGRP	CART
MCH	TRH
Orexin A and B	CRH

■ Insulin

Clinicians who care for diabetics know that when insulin is administered to these patients, weight tends to increase. However, many things change in a diabetic patient who is given insulin, such as reduction in blood glucose and loss of calories through glycosuria.

It has been known for many years that the central administration of insulin into the brain actually decreases feeding. Functional insulin receptors have been identified in many parts of the brain, as have neurons that are sensitive to glucose concentration and changes in glucose concentration, so-called "glucose-sensitive neurons." If insulin is a hormone that increases in response to food intake, it makes sense that it would produce satiety as part of the coordinated response to food ingestion. Recently a transgenic mouse strain was produced where insulin receptors were removed specifically from neuronal cells only (neuron insulin receptor knockout or NIRKO). These mice are obese and infertile although brain development is normal. This experiment provides strong evidence that insulin acts in the brain primarily to reduce food intake and that this effect is important in body weight regulation.

FIGURE 1.

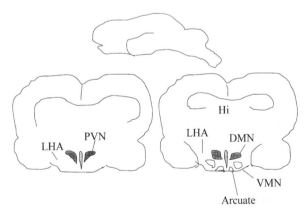

Brain regions involved in the regulation of appetite. The upper panel is a lateral view of a rat brain. The lower panels represent coronal sections through the anterior and posterior hypothalamus. PVN = paraventricular nucleus, LHA = lateral hypothalamic area, Hi = hippocampus, DMN = dorsal medial nucleus, VMN = ventromedial nucleus.

FIGURE 2.

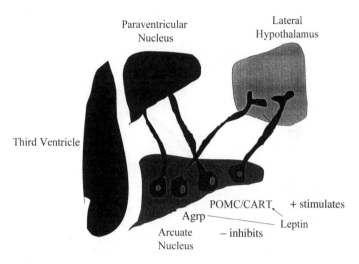

Outline of the neurotransmitter content of neurons that are affected by leptin and project to other hypothalamic nucleii that regulate appetite and body weight. Agrp = agouti related peptide, POMC = pro-opiomelanocortin, CART = cocaine amphetamine related transcript.

■ Summary of Hypothalamic Control of Feeding

As far back as 1954, Elliott Stellar identified a division of labor within the hypothalamus. His early studies demonstrated that lesions of the ventromedial hypothalamus cause weight gain, and that this area was the satiety center. Conversely, lesions of the lateral hypothalamus caused weight loss and he thought this represented a hunger center. Further experiments demonstrated that electrical stimulation of the VMH reduced feeding while electrical stimulation of the LH increased feeding. This added strength to the idea that these two brain centers had opposing functions (Figure 1). More recently, a large number of neuropeptides have been identified that regulate feeding behavior. These peptides can be grouped into those that stimulate feeding (orexigenic) and those that reduce feeding (anorexigenic) (Table 1). Over the last few years the details of the anatomic relationships between relevant brain centers and the neuropeptides that are produced by neurons within these brain centers has been more clearly determined.

It appears that hypothalamic cells activated by leptin interact with two categories of downstream target neurons within the arcuate nucleus. Some of these cells contain NPY and or AGRP, and others contain POMC (Figure 2). These downstream cells then project to the paraventricular nucleus and lateral hypothalamus (Figure 3). In these regions, these cells interact with other downstream effector cells that contain Orexin, MCH, CRH, and TRH. It is now believed that changes in leptin concentration alter positive or negative

FIGURE 3.

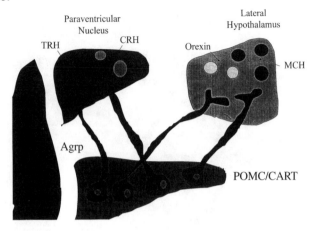

Outline of the neurotransmitter content of neurons downstream from the neurons that are affected by leptin. MCH = melanin concentrating hormone. TRH = thyroptropin-releasing hormone. CHR = corticotropin-releasing hormone.

signals from these brain centers to produce increased or reduced feeding (Figures 4 and 5).

While much of the recent research has focused of the hypothalamus, new areas of research include an extra-hypothalamic site of regulation. ObR is

FIGURE 4.

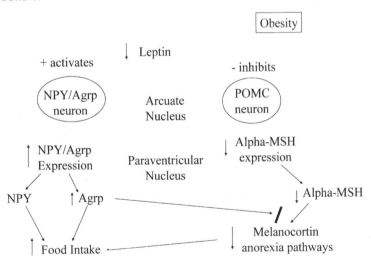

The response of the hypothalamus to a reduction in leptin action. The overall result of these changes is an increase in appetite and weight gain.

FIGURE 5.

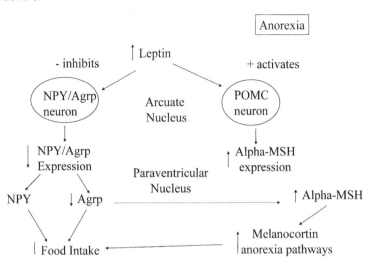

The response of the hypothalamus to an increase in leptin action. The overall result of these changes is a decrease in appetite and weight loss.

expressed in other brain regions including hippocampus and cerebellum. CART is expressed in the spinal cord and orexin in the gastrointestinal tract. Mahogany is expressed in the brain stem and cerebellum, and insulin receptors are present throughout much of the brain. While the function of these regulators of appetite and body weight in these extra-hypothalamic sites is not yet clear, there remain many frontiers for research in the role of these peptides in these extra-hypothalamic locations.

This appears to be a complex system with overlapping signals that both stimulate and inhibit feeding. It is not yet clear which of these pathways are dysfunctional in obese humans and which are the best targets for treatments directed at reducing food intake. However, the advances in our understanding of these regulatory systems are progressing at such a rapid pace that future therapeutic targets hold promise.

In summary, it is reasonable to tell an overweight person that his or her problem with body weight regulation grows out of a dysfunction of a complex biologic system that is poorly adapted to the current environment. In addition, the growing research in the regulation of food intake and body weight offers a promise of new therapeutic agents which may provide effective weight loss for these individuals. In many ways the drug treatment of obesity today is where drug treatment for hypertension was in 1960. There are a few medications that have some effectiveness, but more targeted medications may allow for more effective pharmacologic assistance for obese patients in reducing body weight.

References

1. Schwartz MW, Woods SC, Porte D, Seeley RJ, Baskin DG: Central nervous system control of food intake. Nature 404:661-671, 2000.
2. Elmquist JK, Elias CF, Saper CB: From lesions to leptin: hypothalamic control of food intake and body weight. Neuron 22:221-232, 1999.
3. Barsh G: From Agouti to Pomc—100 years of fat, blonde mice. Nature Medicine 5:984-985, 1999.
4. Cummings DE, Schwartz MW: Melanocortins and body weight: a tale of two receptors. Nature Genetics 26:8-9, 2000.
5. Ahima RS, Flier JS: Leptin. Annu Rev Physiol 62:413-437, 2000.
6. Schwartz, M.W., Mahogany adds color to the evolving story of body weight regulation. Nature Medicine 5:374-375, 1999.

Chapter 22

James O. Hill, PhD, and John C. Peters, PhD

Obesity and the Environment

■ The Obesity Epidemic

Researchers debate about why obesity has reached epidemic proportions in the U.S. and worldwide. The traditional "medical view" of obesity is that some "defect" in physiology leads to an abnormal state of excessive body fat. Many researchers are trying to identify the nature of the physiologic defect, and pharmaceutical companies are searching for drugs that would "fix the problem." An alternative view is that obesity does not represent abnormal physiology, but rather represents a normal physiologic response to the current environment. Whether or not obesity results from normal or abnormal physiology, it is clear that excess body fat contributes to metabolic conditions that often lead to diabetes, heart disease, and other chronic metabolic diseases.[1]

It seems likely that there is some physiologic control of body weight. The best evidence for this is the relative stability of body weight given that almost 1 million calories are ingested each year by an average adult. Without relatively tight control, weight would fluctuate much more than it actually does. Further evidence of the regulation of energy balance is seen with short-term underfeeding and overfeeding experiments. When humans are underfed or overfed for periods of up to 2–3 weeks, there is a compensatory change in energy expenditure to partially counter the change in body weight. After the intervention is stopped, body weight rapidly returns to pre-study levels. However, the ability of this physiological regulatory system is limited since sustained over- or underfeeding will lead to changes in body weight.

It is interesting to examine how this regulatory system likely developed. For most of mankind's history, high levels of physical activity were needed to survive and reproduce (i.e., secure food, security, etc.). Thus, the challenge was getting sufficient food to meet very high energy demands. This may be why there are multiple, redundant systems to facilitate eating. Humans have an innate biologic bias toward eating whenever food is available. Similarly, because high levels of physical activity were required to "get through the day," the system that evolved may have a bias toward resting and conservation of energy when energy expenditure was not urgently needed. These behaviors would have served well in the past, since eating a little extra now and then and resting when there was an opportunity carried little risk and were potentially even beneficial. However, these behaviors do not serve as well in today's environment when food is nearly always available and there is little need to be physically active to subsist and be a productive member of today's society.

Since most of mankind's history was associated more with shortages of food than with excesses of food, the regulatory system likely developed with a bias toward opposing negative energy balance more than positive energy balance. Thus, humans have weaker opposition to overfeeding than to underfeeding. In essence, physiology cannot be relied heavily upon to help avoid obesity. There seems to be no opposition to a "drive" to eat when food is available, the metabolic response to overeating is weak, and no physiologic processes have developed that lead to increase physical activity in response to positive energy balance.

■ The Modern World and Obesity

The current environment in the U.S. is the most conducive to obesity in mankind's history and may "swamp" the ability of the physiologic regulatory system to maintain body weight at a healthy level.[2] The U.S. environment promotes food intake and reduces energy expenditure, leading to a sustained, unidirectional influence on energy balance and resulting in weight gain, as illustrated in Figure 1. Under these conditions, environmental pressures overcome the relatively weak ability of the energy balance regulatory system to oppose positive energy balance and maintain a "healthy" body weight. Sustained positive energy balance leads to increases in body fat and body weight.

Since the body strives to achieve steady-state, this weight gain does not continue indefinitely. As body fat and body weight increase, so does energy expenditure. Total energy expenditure increases because of increases in resting metabolic rate (RMR) due to increased body mass and in the energy expended for physical activity. RMR increases because the positive energy balance produces an increase in body weight that is 20–40% fat-free mass, and RMR increases in proportion to the increase in fat-free mass. The energy expended in physical activity increases because it is energetically more costly to move a larger body than a smaller one. Once body weight has increased sufficiently so that energy expenditure has increased to match energy intake and fat oxidation has increased to meet fat intake, body weight stabilizes and remains stable as long as neither energy intake nor physical activity changes substantially.

■ What Factors in the Modern World Contribute to Obesity?

Factors Affecting Energy Expenditure

Little direct quantitative evidence exists about how factors in the environment contribute to obesity. There is, however, general agreement that the current environment promotes physical inactivity. This is probably occurring in several ways. Most Americans spend most days at work or in school, and both have dramatically reduced in physical activity Very few occupations require substantial amounts of physical activity anymore. Advances in technology have greatly reduced the need for manual labor. Many Americans spend their work day dealing with a computer. Americans no longer pay people to be physically active. Rather, people have to pay (with time or money) to be physically active.[3]

Physical activity in schools has consistently declined over the past decades. Only one state (Illinois) has a requirement for daily physical education. Physical education is disappearing from most schools; where it remains, it often is associated with very little actual physical movement. Similarly, recess periods are being eliminated to provide more opportunity for academic activities.

Most researchers believe that there has been a decline in the amount of physical activity required for daily living over and above declines in the workplace and schools. Dependence on the automobile and advances in technology have made it easy to get through most days with little or no physical activity. People drive to work; use elevators or escalators; sit at computers; send e-mails to the office next door; drive through for food, banking, and dry cleaning; drive home; and spend the evening watching television or surfing the internet. Even stopping by the gym for an hour on the way home does not raise total daily energy expenditure much above resting levels when averaged over the entire day.

Children are especially affected by the increases in technology that have led to a wealth of fun, sedentary activities. They have access to literally hundreds of television channels. They have access to fascinating and stimulating computer games as well as instant access to friends through the internet.

All in all, the American environment encourages a sedentary lifestyle. Physical activity is not necessary anymore in order to get through the day successfully. Unfortunately, most people seem to lack any innate drive to be physically active if physical activity does not serve a useful purpose. If the environment does not require physical activity, people become sedentary. In fact, only about one-third of adults meet the physical activity recommendations of the Surgeon General.[4] The low level of physical activity means that most people have a low total energy expenditure.

Factors Contributing to Increased Energy Intake

Even with a low level of energy expenditure, obesity can be avoided by reducing energy intake appropriately. Unfortunately, the environment also exerts constant pressure to encourage food intake. Some of the factors thought to lead to increased energy intake include a diet high in fat (and high in energy density), large portion sizes, and a wide variety of good tasting, cheap foods. A great deal of research has shown that people eat more total energy when given a diet high in fat than when given a diet low in fat.[5] This may be because high-fat diets are more energy dense (more calories per weight of food) than low-fat diets. Recent research on food intake suggests that people tend to eat about the same volume of food each day, so more energy will be eaten if the food tends to be high in fat and dense. While there have been efforts to reduce the fat content of the U.S. diet, it still remains very high in fat and energy density. Interestingly, there are now efforts to reverse the message that low-fat diets are important for weight management. The best data available suggest that those who achieve low-fat diets are able to avoid weight gain or weight regain after weight loss. Interestingly, data from the U.S. Department of Agriculture show that people who use low-fat food products are able to achieve a diet lower in overall fat than those who do not use these products, but that few people are able to achieve and maintain low fat diets.

A second factor contributing to high energy intake is portion size. Serving large portions of food leads to more total food consumed than when the same food is served in smaller portions. Further, the foods most often served in large portions tend to be those high in fat or energy density.

Finally, the U.S. food supply is characterized by a variety of good tasting, reasonably priced foods. Supermarkets, restaurants, and convenience stores provide a wide choice of food items at competitive prices.

The situation seems relatively simple. The environment facilitates a low energy expenditure and a high energy intake. Under these conditions, obesity is a frequent outcome for many people.

■ What Can We Do?

Cure the Environment

If the environment is making us fat, what can be done to correct the situation? An obvious solution is to change the environment to one that is less obesity-conducive. This is a strategy being discussed more and more within the scientific and public health community. It is difficult to see, however, how the public will ever be able to return the environment to one where most people can maintain a healthy body weight with little effort. This would require an environment requiring a high level of physical activity, yet increases in technology are likely to make physical activity ever less important in achieving productivity. It is unlikely that society will "go back in time" to an environment that makes it difficult to become obese. While there may be ways to alter the environment to make it more supportive of weight maintenance, people must be encouraged to take conscious control of their weight management within the current environment.

Develop Cognitive Skills for Weight Management

One strategy that can be applied immediately is to focus on helping people develop the cognitive skills needed to manage weight within the current obesity-conducive environment. For most of mankind's history, weight management did not require substantial cognitive skills; today, most people who are not paying some attention to their weight are probably gaining weight or are already overweight or obese. Physiology can no longer be relied upon to maintain a healthy body weight. People must learn the skills needed to achieve a balance between energy intake and energy expenditure, and clinicians need to begin building an environment that can help people better manage their body weight.

■ Applying this Information to Obese Patients

Physicians have generally taken a short-term approach to obesity treatment. Patients can make heroic efforts to reduce food intake and to increase physical activity for short periods of time. The typical pattern is for a patient to lose weight (most have done it more than once) but to fail to maintain it. Many obese patients will be unable to maintain a weight loss without significant effort, yet they are not adequately prepared for the effort they will need to maintain their weight.

After weight loss, the patient will have a lower energy requirement than before weight loss. This means that they will have to either eat fewer calories, increase physical activity, or some combination of the above. Furthermore, they will have to do this indefinitely. To achieve weight loss, many patients eat as little as possible and exercise as much as possible. Many people can do this for several weeks or even months, and this may not be a bad strategy to lose weight. However, it is unlikely that many people can continue this indefinitely. Once weight loss is achieved, the challenge of maintenance becomes one of balancing intake with expenditure. It is difficult to do this without easily obtainable, accurate information about energy consumed and energy expended. Here lies a major barrier for patients: obtaining the information needed to achieve energy balance. It is possible to count calories, and indeed this is a marker of successful weight loss maintenance in the National Weight Control Registry, but it is difficult to do with great accuracy. It is much harder to estimate actual energy expenditure. This would involve estimating resting energy expenditure using body weight, accurately quantifying amount and type of physical activity performed, and translating all of this into calories expended. Currently, this task is beyond the capacity of most patients.

The National Weight Control Registry subjects are successful because they carefully monitor body weight and are able to adjust intake and/or physical activity patterns to keep weight constant (see chapter 17). This is probably not the best avenue for success, since often substantial positive energy balance exists by the time significant weight changes occur. A better strategy advocates having sufficient information about energy ingested and energy expended to identify periods of positive energy balance before body weight increases.

The key to treating obesity is helping to prevent weight regain after weight loss and to teach people how to understand and achieve energy balance. Some environmental changes are needed to do this more effectively.

For example, nutrient information exists for many food products but not for food consumed in restaurants. It is hard to provide information about energy expended but a new generation of pedometers provides useful feedback on energy expended. At the same time the environment must change to one that provides information about energy intake and energy expenditure, patients need to learn about energy balance and about how to match intake with expenditure.

■ Incentives for Achieving Energy Balance

For many people, it will take considerable effort to achieve energy balance by cognitive means. These people need appropriate incentives (and possibly disincentives) to aid in their success.

It is unlikely that people will tolerate, on principle, rationing of the food supply to limit intake, notwithstanding the tremendous social and economic consequences of such a policy. Likewise, it is unlikely society would willingly choose to adopt measures that regulate access to sedentary-behavior–promoting technologies, given the devastating impact on productivity that would occur. Opportunities must be provided for people to eat healthier and become more active, and people must make use of these opportunities.

Years of research in public health have made it apparent that simply providing people with knowledge and skills alone is insufficient motivation for behavior change. Often, the negative health effects of poor behavior choices and the health benefits of positive behavior change will not be realized until years later, and immediate gratification is difficult to overcome. Given this dynamic, encouraging people to make healthier choices needs to be tied to some immediate, meaningful benefit.

Critics of the food industry have suggested using taxes on foods high in fat and calories like snack foods, fast foods, and carbonated soft drinks to raise money to pay for marketing and advertising of fruits and vegetables. This assumes, of course, that increased advertising of these inherently low-calorie foods will increase their consumption and presumably limit intake of more calorie-dense foods. Unfortunately, there is little evidence for this desired effect, and there is concern that such taxes would disproportionately burden individuals of lower socioeconomic status who are more likely to suffer from food insecurity (persistent concern over the availability of food).

Alternatively, incentives should be offered (e.g., lower taxes, state or federal support) to school districts, restaurants, and other food purveyors to offer portion sizes and food selections that meet USDA guidelines. Restaurants and cafeterias should be given incentives for labeling food portions to indicate the calorie content and proportion of total daily energy needs, making it easier for people to select a reasonable portion size. Individuals could be offered incentives for selecting recommended foods and portions. Making the healthiest meal the best value (e.g., most nutrients per dollar, biggest toy, etc.) may increase demand. For children, simply having a voice in the process may promote healthier behaviors. Some schools have tried letting students select what food choices will be offered in the cafeteria from among a variety of only healthy choices. The students were able to find healthy items that they liked, and because they were empowered to choose, they felt ownership of the outcome. The schools documented a 60% decrease in plate waste, meaning the kids were actually eating the healthy food.

The same principles can be applied to incentives/disincentives for promoting physical activity. Unlike the case for food, no one has yet suggested that a tax on labor-saving devices or transportation in order to discourage their use or to use the revenue to promote activity. Why not make people pay a toll to use the escalator instead of the stairs or pay to take the elevator for only a few floors? What about taxing remote controls or increasing the tax on gasoline to generate revenue to promote public transit or to build more safe walkways? Since our society has embraced numerous labor-saving and time-saving technologies as a basic strategy for increasing total productivity, it seems unlikely that restrictive or punitive measures would be adopted to discourage sedentary behavior. It seems more reasonable to explore incentives for making the environment more friendly toward activity and for encouraging more active lifestyles.

To that end, tax and other incentives could be offered to developers to include safe walkways and prominent stair access in all new developments and in urban renewal projects. Large employers could receive incentives to offer facilities (e.g., trails, showers, exercise facilities) and time for employees to engage in physical activity at work. Individuals should be encouraged to use these facilities by offering what is most valuable to them, time, in return for their investment in health. Some employers already give workers additional paid vacation if they take a yearly physical fitness test and show that they continue to improve on or meet targets for fitness. Employers adopting these programs report fewer worker sick days and greater job satisfaction, which adds up to greater productivity.

Even children can be given incentives to be more physically active, if the incentive is something of value to them. For example, inexpensive physical activity monitors (pedometers and accelerometers) are now available to record physical activity throughout the day. Parents could allow children to spend time at the computer or in front of the TV based on the amount of physical activity the child gets during the day. Thus the parent would be able to regulate access to sedentary activity, while the child controls how much time is spent in these activities.

None of these interventions alone will be successful in eradicating obesity and restoring energy balance on a population-wide scale. Because obesity is so complex and involves myriad causal factors in our society, it is likely that we will only be able to turn back the tide with a multitude of small, unidirectional changes in the environment that support healthier eating and more active living.

References

1. National Institutes of Health: Clinical guidelines on the identification, evaluation, and treatment of overweight and obesity in adults—the Evidence Report. Obes Res 6 (Suppl 2) 51S-210S, 1998.
2. Hill JO, Peters JC: Environmental contributions to the obesity epidemic. Science 280:1371, 1998.
3. Philipson T: The world-wide growth in obesity: an economic research agenda. Health Economics 10:1-7, 2001.
4. Hill, JO, Peters JC: The impact of diet composition on energy and nutrient balance. Progress in Obesity Reseearch 7:385-392, 1996.
5. French SA, Story M, Jeffery RW: Environmental Influences on eating and physical activity. Annual Review of Public Health 22:309-335, 2001.
6. Kennedy E, Bowman S: Assessment of the effect of fat-modified foods on diet quality in adults, 19 to 50 years, using data from the Continuing Survey of Food Intake by Individuals. J Am Diet Assoc 101(4):455-460, 2001.

INDEX

Page numbers in **boldface type** indicate complete chapters.